THE AROMATHERAPY

The Aromatherapy Workshop

Nicole Perez

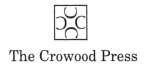

The Crowood Press

First published in 2000 by
The Crowood Press Ltd
Ramsbury, Marlborough
Wiltshire SN8 2HR

This impression 2000

British Library Cataloguing-in-Publication Data
A catalogue record for this book is available from
the British Library.

ISBN 1 86126 256 6

Dedication
To my very special daughter, Tara Woolnough.

Acknowledgements
Thank you very much to Alexandra House for her
big help in researching, typing and proof-reading
this book.

Special thanks for help with writing the book to
Anita Lewis, Deborah Nix, Tara and Keith Wool-
nough, Hilary Marks, Carol Horrigan, Marlgozata
Pawlaczik, Barbara Keen, Roger Dyer and Elaine
Arthey.

Also thanks for help along the way to Linda
Harness, Mai Dunphy, Ivan Everett, Hilary
Deeble-Rogers, Margaret Canning, Jeremy Bewley
and to everyone else not listed here; the list would
be long.

Typefaces used: Galliard and Franklin Gothic.

Typeset and designed by
D & N Publishing
Membury Business Park, Lambourn Woodlands
Hungerford, Berkshire.

Printed and bound in Great Britain by Bookcraft (Bath) Ltd, Midsomer Norton, Somerset

Contents

The Garden

A long time ago, before Science and Art were well established among men, there lived a Master Gardener. He knew all about the nutritious and medicinal qualities of plants. He also knew about the 'herb of longevity' and lived for many hundreds of years. He taught successive generations of people, all over the world, how to plant and maintain a garden.

In one place, he planted a wonderful garden and taught the people how to care for it. However, people soon took the garden's beauty for granted, becoming accustomed to seeing the many plants blossom every year. Over time, they forgot that some were grown from seeds that needed collecting, others were grown from cuttings, while others needed special watering care, and so on.

After a long period of neglect, the wonderful garden reverted to being wild, and the beautiful plants became indistinguishable from the invading weeds. Because people had forgotten the original garden, they now started to look upon this garden as the best garden there could be ...

Inspired from a traditional Chisti story called *The Garden*

Nature is proficient and creates all sorts, plants or beings. However, it is up to each one of us to cultivate our inner virtues so that the garden of our lives and in it our good health and happiness can flourish naturally.

CHAPTER 1
Heal: To Make Whole and Healthy ...

Since the awakening of public interest in the 'new natural therapies' in the mid-1980s, Aromatherapy has proved to be the most popular natural answer to stress and stress-related problems.

It is also an established fact that Aromatherapy is particularly useful when dealing with the treatment of minor ailments. One of the reasons why Aromatherapy oils are often a first choice for treating such ailments is simply that they work. Furthermore, in my experience as a practitioner and teacher, I have met many women who mourn the loss of the knowledge of natural remedies or cures which was handed down from mother to daughter through the generations. This longing for 'old-fashioned' medicine reflects the growing concern of many people about the long-term effects of synthetic pharmaceutical remedies. The interesting thing is that even the pharmacists themselves are now recognizing this need for a more gentle medicine, which is reflected in the many herbal products currently available in most big chemists and superstores.

It may be asked, however, what the real therapeutic benefits of Aromatherapy are and what aspects of it are just a 'fad'. There is no doubt that there is a fashionable aspect to Aromatherapy, but this has more to do with the cosmetics industry and the related media than with the caring and truly healing work of the professional Aromatherapist. Aromatherapy is often described as a truly holistic treatment as it works both psychologically and physiologically, as all the essential oils have certain recognized therapeutic properties. Having said that, the detailed therapeutic effects of Aromatherapy are not clear-cut, and although one may see good results and a marked improvement in health, further research is needed to be able to demonstrate in a scientific manner why and how such healing took place.

Something that is a bit misleading for lay people is that Aromatherapy is often presented as being an ancient therapy which has existed for thousands of years. Indeed, aromatic plants and their uses have been known to mankind for centuries and there are many indications in ancient texts from Egypt and India that it existed there as a refined science. However, Aromatherapy as it is practised today did not really come into existence until the turn of the twentieth century when R.H. Gattefosse, a French perfumer and chemist, undertook the huge task of researching the chemical properties of essential oils. As a result of this work, he was able to lay down the foundations of a scientifically based therapy using essential oils, and in the process gave Aromatherapy its name. His findings have since been widely used by many for the further development of Aromatherapy.

Gattefosse was a man with a vision, who perceived that the power of essential oils not only restored the body but also could 'cure' the mind through interacting with the sense of smell and the central nervous system. He held the restorative powers of essential oils in great esteem and realized their therapeutic potential; he also held the view that natural substances used in their *totum* were more efficient and safer that the use of isolated constituents. He therefore believed that individual chemicals should be confined for use in pharmacy, possibly combined with other pharmaceutical chemicals.

There are currently many pharmaceutical remedies containing natural chemical constituents extracted from plants. Pharmaceutical remedies are generally made with the aim of optimizing the strength of a remedy, enabling it to work more specifically and with a more rapid action than herbal remedies. Herbal remedies are known to take some time to take effect and are not always the best choice when dealing with a health crisis. As a result, they have been marginalized as a possible form of medical treatment. What is beginning to become apparent, however, is that the human body does not easily process many of the pharmaceutical remedies and although these may have had a successful effect in relieving symptoms, the after-effects in many instances may leave the body with secondary problems, for example when steroid creams are used for certain skin disorders. Sometimes they work well, but sometimes the complaint keeps on getting worse. Many practitioners, including some GPs, are aware of these problems and are trying to educate patients to take better care of their health and avoid the inappropriate use of medicine.

Aromatherapy works in a different way as the natural essences found in aromatic plants, the essential oils, seem to be more adaptable when interacting with the human body than their artificially manufactured chemical counterparts. The scope of activity of essential oils is very wide and their efficacy often comes as a surprise. To give an idea

of the range of benefits they offer, here are some of their general therapeutic properties. Many of them are antiseptics, bactericides, expectorants, anxyolitics, tonics, stimulants, relaxants, sedatives and calmatives. More curiously, some of the essential oils are known to stimulate emotional reactions such as the release of fear or anger. Even the intimate life of a person can benefit as the essential oils have earned a reputation for increasing the libido in people suffering from low sexual drive, although unfortunately this has resulted in the exaggeration of their aphrodisiac powers.

To come back to the development of Aromatherapy during the twentieth century, the interest of the pioneers of Aromatherapy such as Gattefosse and Dr J. Valnet (Dr Valnet, now in retirement, was a French Army doctor who, during the 1950s successfully used aromatic preparations on the wounded. After leaving the Army in 1959, he concentrated on researching the therapeutic effects of essential oils and wrote many books, one of them *Aromatherapie, traitement des maladies par les essences des plants* became the first Aromatherapy textbook and is now available in English.) focused mostly on the activity of essential oils on the body when taken orally. Valnet in particular used essential oils as a substitute for pharmaceutical remedies and obtained remarkable results. This is fine for some health crises, but essential oils are quite powerful as they are very concentrated and they too have their limitations. However, there is another approach to using essential oils apart from ingestion. Studies carried out during the last fifteen years have found that one of the most direct routes for the absorption of essential oils into the body is through inhalation. Inhaling an essential oil will result in a small amount reaching the lungs with the air from the breath and becoming absorbed into the bloodstream as the exchange of gases takes place. Although only a minute amount of essential oil may be reaching various body tissues, it is believed that even such a tiny amount has the capacity to 'energize' body cells and thus strengthen the 'terrain'. (Terrain: the internal environment or ground in the body which promotes good health or illnesses.) In other words, strengthening the body's cellular environment helps the weakened tissues to recover. As stated above, some of the essential oils contain chemical components that have distinct properties such as antiseptic or antibacterial, and it is the activity of these components that can counteract the destructive effects of microorganisms responsible for some diseases.

But the 'miracle' of essential oils does not stop there. Equally important is the psychological effect that the smells of essential oils have on people when interacting with the olfactory system. This has already been briefly highlighted and will be fully explained later in this book.

Some people question the validity and the safety of replacing allopathic remedies with natural remedies such as essential oils. The biochemistry which takes place in the human body is an endless maze of complex processes that assemble and disassemble chemical substances for the purpose of maintaining and facilitating the growth of body tissues. These processes are ultimately there for the benefit of the whole organism. There is a relationship of affinity between chemicals from plants and chemicals found in the human body as they both originate from carbon.

This relationship is important as the human body often seems to be more able to deal with chemical substances that have occurred naturally, as they are likely to be readily eliminated once they have performed their job. At this point, clarification is needed regarding what is meant by natural remedies being better for the body. Natural does not necessarily mean safe. Essential oils need to be from reliable sources and must be administered correctly to ensure that no harm is caused to the body cells by misuse. They are at their most efficacious when the natural compounds within them are allowed to remain intact so as to interact in synergy with each other. Further to the above considerations, there is also the actual treatment: the environment in which it takes place, whether the approach is holistic, or whether a more clinical approach is required. Who the therapist is, is also important. All of these are parts of what constitute the conditions for healing. Most people today understand that the holistic approach to health means that health problems are looked at in the context of a person's 'whole' life – mind, body and spirit need to be in a state of equilibrium with each other. If one aspect becomes unbalanced, it can lead to physical or mental illness.

THE HOLISTIC APPROACH TO HEALING THE MIND AND BODY

When looking into the causes of 'unwellness', some of the most important considerations are a person's lifestyle and their degree of self-contentment. Here are some of the factors considered to lead to better health and treatment:

Beneficial Factors	Negative Factors
Balanced Lifestyle Adequate rest and recreation; regular exercise; a healthy diet; ability to relax.	*Strenuous Lifestyle* Not enough sleep; too much work; no breaks or holidays; burdened by responsibility.

This leads to:

9

Helpful Factors for a Successful Treatment

Positive Factors	*Negative Factors*
• A warm and friendly environment.	• An imposing and over-sterile environment.
• Relaxed relationship between patient/ therapist.	• An impersonal relationship.
• A caring approach.	• An over-clinical and dissociative approach.
• A thorough clinical knowledge of Aromatherapy, used with sensitivity and intuition when deciding on a treatment.	• Adhering too rigidly to formulae and the rules of practice, thereby failing to treat the client as an individual.

COMPLEMENTARY APPROACH OR ALLOPATHIC MEDICINE?

All should have the right to choose both.

Choosing Aromatherapy as a Means of Treatment

The same questions are frequently asked regarding the true benefits of Aromatherapy. This is caused by the many contradictions to be found in the current Aromatherapy literature. There is confusion regarding the properties of essential oils, and some books give the impression that many ailments can be easily treated at home. Common sense needs to be brought into play – for example, if a patient is in exclusive need of surgery, then chemicals are not going to solve the problem. Consideration must be given to how much pain or worry the problem has caused and how long it has been going on. Has it been correctly diagnosed and would medical treatment be more suitable before embarking on self-treatment? Is it a simple problem or would a professional Aromatherapist provide a better assessment and results?

The really wonderful thing about Aromatherapy is that one does not need to be ill to reap the benefits from a treatment. The essential oils have remarkable re-vitalizing properties, and for the healthy person their use can certainly help to keep the doctor away. For the less healthy person, Aromatherapy can provide a non-aggressive natural treatment which can be used as a supportive physical and psychological aid to another form of treatment.

The question is, therefore, what can Aromatherapy do for you?

SOME OF THE MAIN BENEFITS OF AROMATHERAPY

First Aid of Minor Ailments

Aromatherapy is very useful in the home for things such as cuts, grazes, small burns, headaches, sprains and aches.

Calming Severe Stress Symptoms and Acute Anxiety

The gentle tranquillizing properties of some of the essential oils can calm stress symptoms such as an irregular or rapid heart beat, light-headedness, shallow breathing and so on.

Creating a Positive Mood

Aromatherapy can uplift the mind, altering the way we feel and also helping to change our attitudes towards ourselves or what is upsetting us.

CLINICAL BENEFITS OF AROMATHERAPY

Essential Oils and the Immune System

Aromatherapy promotes a quicker and heightened response and can work alongside conventional medicine such as powerful antiseptics or antibiotics.

Anti-Infectious Therapeutic Properties

The use of essential oils can prevent further infection where there is an organ injury, for example, MRSA (one of the 'superbugs' currently responsible for wound infections caught in hospital, which do not respond to normal antibiotic treatments), gangrene or broken bones. Vaporization, inhalation and direct application can help to fight viral and bacterial infections. The use of oils helps to promote good blood circulation – some of the essential oils are vasoconstrictive and can therefore help in strengthening the venous system.

General and Specific Muscular and Skeletal Problems

Essential oils are natural anti-spasmodics and analgesics and are a great help with aches, pains and general tension. The combination of skilful massage and the myorelaxing therapeutic properties of the oils can ease any restriction caused by recent or old injuries.

Where there is inflammation in the muscles or joints, the anti-inflammatory properties of essential oils can provide efficient pain relief and speed the recovery process. Many essential oils have therapeutic properties which tend to speed up the healing of fractured bones and in reversing the damage to joints caused by diseases such as arthritis.

Improving Breathing and Respiration

Shallow breathing is part of the price we have to pay for living in a polluted and stressful environment. Essential oils can be used as expectorants, emollients and respiratory antiseptics and have many properties that help ease respiratory ailments. Inhalation is the quickest way for essential oils to get into the system and tackle viral infections. Inhalation also deepens the breath and can regulate spasmodic respiration caused by chronic bronchitis or asthma.

Fighting Urinary Infections

The urinary system can also benefit from the therapeutic properties of essential oils as they help fight infections and can calm inflammatory symptoms.

Promoting Good Digestion

The action of essential oils can increase the action of peristalsis and facilitate digestion and excretion.

Improving the Skin

Again, the versatility of essential oils becomes self-evident when dealing with skin problems, as repair can occur very rapidly with their use. They can be beneficial not only in the treatment of oily or dry skin, but also for rashes, burns, dermatitis or infected skin.

Restoring the Body Energies

Aromatherapy restores stamina, in the long run increasing the level of energy and restoring the body from accumulated fatigue.

Use in Psychosomatic Conditions

Contrary to an earlier belief this century that 'the human body is a machine with spare parts', it is now evident 'that the human body is not a machine and has very few parts to spare, if any at all'. The human organism is constantly trying to adapt and rebalance itself through homeostasis and any treatment which is too fierce, even when there is a life-threatening condition, might not lead to proper healing as it puts the body in a state of trauma.

The patients themselves may also be in a state of shock from the news of their illness, something that will hinder proper healing during treatment. Natural therapies such as Aromatherapy can be particularly helpful in dealing with the emotional overload which often prevents proper physical healing.

Natural Consequences

In 1653, the great English herbalist, Nicholas Culpeper, published his classic encyclopaedia, listing the properties of many hundreds of plants and the use of their oils. This work, *The Physical Directory,* was so popular that it has been republished in forty-one editions and is still in print today. 'I doubt not', he wrote, 'but for every disease, there is in nature a sever-all symple.'

If illness is a natural phenomenon, then so – he believed – must be the cure.

CHAPTER 2
The Holistic Viewpoint

Health matters have naturally been of continuous concern to humanity, and many famous physicians throughout history have contributed to the knowledge of medicine that prevails nowadays. There are certain 'gaps' which exist in the practice of modern medicine, such as the prevention of illness or the maintenance of good health and allowing for a period of recovery once the health crisis has been effectively dealt with. Neglect of these areas of healthcare has resulted in a large number of people not being aware that they should follow a certain amount of restraint regarding diet or physical activities and even work. Too frequently, patients are discharged from treatment with inadequate aftercare advice.

In ancient China, the Imperial physician would have been put to death if any members of the Imperial family had fallen ill, as his job was to ensure that the rulers stayed in top condition until the end of their lives. Indeed, the Chinese have a reputation for living very long lives and this alone should say something about their knowledge of health matters. The revival of ancient medicine in its modern, complementary form is in part dedicated to the continuation of healthy living. As my own GP once told me, no treatment is ever going to be as good as not needing that treatment in the first place. It is my belief that complications and recurrences of illnesses are the result of too little attention being paid to the prevention of ill health or to the convalescence period that is necessary after a successful treatment so that the body can regain its full functioning capacity.

Not enough emphasis is put on educating the public in how they can help prevent ill health. These days, conventional medical practitioners rarely have the time or resources to deal with any stress their patients may experience, and despite successfully treating many illnesses there are not enough resources to address the issue of convalescence and proper recovery. Aromatherapy can provide a range of healing outcomes that will address the problems of both the mind and body.

The practice of Aromatherapy has many facets, one of which is the clinical aspect. This clinical facet offers us the possibility of treating specific ailments just as one would be using conventional medicines, but with the extra promise that the underlying cause may be resolved too. There is always a need to tackle the psychodynamic forces that lie behind many health crises, as these are likely to be responsible for some of the physiological imbalances. Aromatherapy can therefore be put to use as an aid to allopathic medicine or as a therapy in its own right.

As already mentioned in the first chapter, many modern pharmaceutical remedies still contain ingredients extracted from plants, which are then processed in a certain way so as to optimize their strength. It is becoming increasingly apparent that there is more than one answer to many medical problems. Safety in medicine is the primary concern and one of the important factors in healing is that products should be easily eliminated once the body has taken what it requires from them. If the products are not broken down and excreted properly, they continue being active and may prevent the body from generating its own healing power in the future. The traditional approach to health for centuries has been that if the body is sick, the symptoms should be considered in their context and the ill person rather than just the symptoms should be treated. It is also accepted that each illness has its own course of development and often the way to help recovery is not to 'stop' the problems but rather to speed up the passage of the illness. The body's organs also need fortifying and their health is increased when excretion of waste products is facilitated. This is still at the core of increased immune activity and diuretics, sudorifics, mucolytics, diaphoretics and carminative remedies are extremely important in medicine. Further to this, a healthy diet and proper rest will also help in strengthening the whole organism.

So, what is the secret of a successful and holistic Aromatherapy treatment? It is a combination of sound scientific and practical knowledge combined with observation and intuitive skills. Without all of these it is not possible to assess the situation and decide what course of treatment is most appropriate.

Assessing problems correctly and prescribing the best remedies for them is always a difficult task and relies on the personal ability of the therapist, the therapist's attitude towards illness and the quality of the relationship between the therapist and client. The client needs to feel able to trust the therapist in order to be receptive to the more subtle aspects of the treatment. Nor is the application of Aromatherapy straightforward, as different people will have different responses to treatments. To work efficiently, the treatment *must* be safe. Essential oils may be natural, but they are also extremely concentrated and powerful and the choice and dosage of these oils must be carefully controlled.

Consequently, it is unwise to treat ailments without a good knowledge of the workings of the body and a full understanding of the activity of essential oils. This is not necessarily wrong, but it would be a bit like walking in the dark in an unknown landscape; it is potentially dangerous. Natural medicine is not any different from allopathic medicine in that it also has its dangers and limitations.

One therefore has to tread carefully on known grounds before embarking upon the treatment of persons suffering from complicated or unusual illnesses. Even when essential oils are known to relieve some of the symptoms, a good knowledge of a disease at the outset of treatment, combined with a logical categorization of the effects of the remedies, is essential.

An Aromatherapy treatment can be applied in various ways. All the different approaches are valid as they represent different situations and conditions.

Applications of Aromatherapy	Different Approaches
i Topical	Direct application on the skin.
ii First aid	The best application to have immediate effect.
iii First-time treatment	To begin gently and not put the organism under attack.
iv Holistic approach	Must include an assessment based on the physical and emotional life of a client.

16

DEFINITION OF HOLISTIC AROMATHERAPY

1. Treatments which address physiological and physical problems. These include massage, inhalation, rubbing, compresses, baths, ointments and creams.
2. Treatments which address psychological, psychosomatic or anxiety problems. These include olfactory stimulation to achieve psychological out comes. A study of olfaction, scents and traditional associations of perfumes, combined with a knowledge of personality traits, is necessary to understand the effects of this form of therapy upon people.

It must also be stressed that a knowledge of the patient's medical history is part of every consultation and is necessary to a successful treatment. A history of current and past states of health helps to establish patterns of illness. Stress can also be assessed on a scale of ten and monitored weekly to see if the health problems diminish when there is less stress. The posture and general outlook or temperament of clients can be also noted, as these may increase stress in times of pressure. Signs of excessive sensitivity, timidity or anxiety should also be recorded, as these are often at the root of many psychosomatic illnesses. Aromatherapy is known to have a positive effect on such underlying factors. Other factors which can increase stress levels are pollution, hyperventilation and no proper relaxation. Stress will often show as sudden changes of moods and acute irritability or depression.

The chart below shows the moods or attitudes which can have a positive or negative effect upon our general well being.

THE ROOT OF PSYCHOSOMATIC AILMENTS

The process of growing up consists of a myriad of experiences, both small and large, which form many of the body's reflexes that maintain health. It starts at birth when we have to take in our first breath; already a new reflex has been implemented. It progresses with suckling milk and later learning to digest solid food. While this happens, other experiences are also taking place, such as learning to hold our heads straight, crawling, standing, walking, running, dancing and so on. By the time we reach twenty years of age, we will have acquired the majority of the involuntary reflexes that give us certain preconditioned responses to many situations. However, human beings, like other living organisms, also need to evolve on an individual basis as well as a collective one. There are some modern medical scientists who have come to regard illnesses and disorders as a form of evolution, in that they force us to develop new survival skills. These scientists claim that if people have been ill and are left with some disabilities from it, they are also left with valuable and important new experiences. They should be praised for their body having

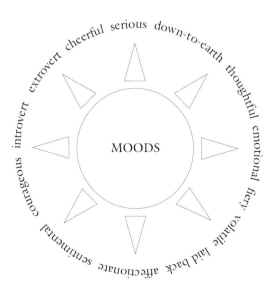

adapted to this new situation, rather than feeling that their body or themselves have failed in some way.

Shock and Trauma

Amongst many healers it is an accepted fact that the effects of shock and trauma tend to remain in the body long after the initial event and can create involuntary muscle tension, causing obstacles to the flow of nervous energy which in turn may lead to illness or repeated unpleasant experiences. Trauma or shock can easily become automatic responses and reflexes, manifesting as allergies, postural weaknesses, inhibition of metabolic processes, problems with the assimilation of nutrients, respiratory difficulties, and so on. Once responses have become reflexes, they are controlled by the autonomic nervous system and therefore occur involuntarily. Sometimes these problems cannot be rectified, but in many instances Aromatherapy offers the chance to go deeper into the psyche, bypassing the current response and resetting the body's functions in a more harmonious way. Illnesses are treated as imbalances in the body. To restore that balance, it is necessary to restore emotional and physiological homeostasis.

CHAPTER 3

Botanical Origins of Aromatic Plants

The Very Secret Life of Aromatic Plants

When wild lavender saw the trials and torments suffered by other flowers, pressed in bunches or abandoned in contempt, she said 'How lucky I am not to be a decoration in a flower bed. Contrary to the custom with other flowers, nature has me growing far from streams. I like isolated places. I am never one of a crowd.
Sheikh Izzidin Al-Muquaddisi (1280)

BOTANY AND THERAPEUTICS

Plant Origins and their Environmental and Therapeutic Characteristics

It all begins in the natural environment in which we live. Just as we have had to adapt to geographical and climatic challenges, so have plants. Like us, they have evolved over thousands of years. Some species, having existed in a similar form since antiquity, have earned themselves a place in traditional folk medicine for their beneficial and therapeutic properties. Meanwhile, some plants, due to the recent new approach to science and medicine, are just beginning to be investigated with great hopes. One such plant is the Yew tree, *Taxus brevifolia*, one of whose chemical components, taxol, a nitrogenous diterpene, is currently the subject of intense study as a possible anti-cancer drug.

Fragrant Plants and their Therapeutic Essential Oils

In the botanical world there are thousands of plants which have medicinal properties, although not all of them contain the fragrant essential oils which are used in Aromatherapy.

Many textbooks on Aromatherapy already include botanical data concerning the origins and classification of the aromatic plants involved. This botanical information helps to define the most suitable uses of particular essential oils. For example, most essential oils extracted from trees belonging to the large family of the *Pinaceae* will exhibit, to varying degrees, therapeutic properties beneficial to the respiratory and excretory system.

A plant's habitat is fundamental to the properties it will develop, as plants derive much of their tendencies from the following:

- The soil, for example what types of minerals are predominant.
- The climate: whether temperate, tropical or polar, for example.
- How much sun or water they receive.
- The prevailing weather conditions.
- The weather condition in the particular year that the plants were collected.
- The particular plant species.

Other factors which affect directly the quality of essential oils are:

- The methods of collecting the plants and extracting their essential oils.
- Their storage and lifespan.

All of the above are contributing factors to the type of chemical make-up, quality and purity of the essential oil produced and its efficiency in therapeutic terms.

The therapeutic properties of essential oils are multiple and diverse, and to the many newcomers and students of Aromatherapy it is not always clear how this data fits in with the practical application of the therapy. Some therapeutic properties are found in certain botanical species of aromatic plants but do not exist in the essential oils. Some therapeutic properties belong to an individual or group of chemical components found in an essential oil, but these may account for only some of an essential oil's benefits.

This is because some of the chemicals work in synergy, reinforcing each other's properties and thus creating a wider spectrum of therapeutic benefits, making it difficult to know what particular chemical is responsible for what particular effect. However, what really interests us here are the benefits that can be derived from certain aromatic plants. Such benefits have been the subject of study for centuries. 'Systematic botany' really began to be notated in the 1700s and has been evolving ever since. Many of the

rules that were laid down then on how to allocate the right place to the right plant and to name it are still in use. Early in the nineteenth century, a more specialized branch of botany called 'pharmacognosy', appeared. Pharmacognosy is mostly concerned with the use of substances obtained from natural sources, mainly plants, and how they can be used to make remedies and aids in the treatment of disease. It concentrates more particularly on the study of the chemicals responsible for the therapeutic effects, and its purpose is to be as precise and accurate as possible. Phytochemistry, the study of a plant's chemicals, is a specialized branch of pharmacy and it has grown in importance now that the general public is increasingly turning away from synthetic drugs towards 'natural herbal cures' to treat many health problems. Today, it is not just the medical herbalist or the Aromatherapy student who has to learn the therapeutic benefits and chemical tendencies of plants, but pharmacy students too, as mainstream pharmacy incorporates more and more plant-derived products.

Presently, there is some disparity in Aromatherapy books regarding certain aromatic plants and which family they may belong to. In Aromatherapy, only a fraction of the complete botanical classification is needed, as the purpose of knowing the botanical name of a plant is to ascertain as precisely as possible whether the plant and more particularly its essential oil(s) have particular therapeutic or toxic tendencies.

How Botanical Names of Particular Plants are Determined

Botany is the study of the biological life of plants. It involves all aspects of plant life, from their origins on the planet to the preferred habitats of plants, climatic adaptation, migration, regeneration habits, system of propagation or reproduction, structure, chemical content of the plant and its volatile oil, toxicity or therapeutic benefits of the latter and any already existing historical names. As can be seen, amongst scientific studies botany constitutes an extensive subject made up of a very complex system of division and subdivision for the classification of all known plants and their appropriate naming. The word 'botany' itself is derived from the ancient Greek word for 'grass' or 'herb', although of course today the subject includes all plant forms.

Plant Classification and General Naming

A definite hierarchy for plant classification is used, ranging from the larger groupings down to the smaller subdivisions, in the order listed here:

- Divisions, classes, subclasses, orders, suborders, family, subfamilies, tribes, genera, species and varieties.

Latin is the language that forms the basis for the naming of plants, and the ending of the Latin name gives a clue as to its position in the division process. For example, orders of plants always end in *ales*, but most botanical family and subfamily names end in *aceae*, particularly, the ones named or renamed in recent times. Sometimes, plants can have a slightly different ending, indicating a specific divisional placement within the hierarchy of their botanical main family. However, there are still a number of plants that have been traditionally known under certain family names and that do not fall under this system of naming.

Classification and naming of botanical plants is under the guidance of the international code of botanical nomenclature; however, despite this, what one botanist may consider as a family another may regard as a subfamily. For example, camomile is classified under the family of the *Compositae*, the largest of the flowering plant families with about 900 genera and more than 13,000 species. In some of the more recent Aromatherapy books, however, camomile has been placed in the family of the *Asteraceae*, a subfamily of the *Compositae*. Only the botanical names of the family, subfamily (if relevant) and the genus/variety of each aromatic plant from which essential oils are extracted have been listed in the botanical table in this book.

Variations in the names of plants can exist among books about Aromatherapy, such as *Umbelliferae* also being listed as *Apiaceae*, *Labiatae* as *Lamiaceae*, *Pinaceae* as *Abietaceae*. The second of each category shows more precision in the suborder.

Botanical Families			
Botanical Class and Name	Specific Plants	Geographical Occurrence and Features	General Therapeutic Activity
ANNONACEAE (family of the Magnoliales order)	Ylang-Ylang	These small trees grow particularly in the Philippines, Madagascar and Comoros Island.	Cardio-regulator, expectorant, anti-depressant and stress-related disorders, anti-acneic, sedative.

continued overleaf

Botanical Families *continued*			
Botanical Class and Name	Specific Plants	Geographical Occurrence and Features	General Therapeutic Activity
BURSERACEAE	Frankincense, Myrrh, Elemi	Tropical shrubs found in Arabia, North Africa and Tropical America.	Antiseptic, healing, anti-inflammatory.
COMPOSITAE Asteraceae	Camomile, Tarragon, Calendula, Arnica, Tagetes	Largest family of flowering plants, growing in temperate to subtropical climates.	Mild sedative, antiseptic, anti-inflammatory, anti-spasmodic, vulnerary.
CONIFERAE Pinaceae; Cupressaceae	Juniper, Cypress, Pine, Cedar	Most ancient botanical family. Mostly trees with needles, abundant in the northern hemisphere, spreading south to Indonesia and Australia.	Anti-fungal, rubefacient, tonic, respiratory, antiseptic, anti-spasmodic.
GERANIACEAE Genus: *Pelargonium*	Scented Geranium: Lemon Geranium, Rose Geranium, etc.	Mediterranean, northern Africa and subtropical zones: Réunion, Madagascar and Guinea.	Astringent, haemostatic, antiseptic, endocrine system, anti-spasmodic, analgesic, anti-depressant, healing for all skin problems.
GRAMINEAE	*Cymbopogon*: Citronella, Lemon Grass, Palmarosa. *Andropogon*: Vetivert	Fragrant grasses from tropical and subtropical zones: India, Madagascar and the West Indies.	Stomachic, sudorific, carminative, vulnerary and diaphoretic. Parasiticide and insecticide.
ILLICIACEAE (Magnoliaceae)	Star aniseed	An evergreen tree from south-west China, Vietnam, eastern North America and the West Indies.	Nervous stimulant, digestive, carminative, aperitive, antiseptic, expectorant.
JASMINACEAE	Jasmine	Tropical and subtropical zones.	Anti-depressant, astringent.

Botanical Families *continued*			
Botanical Class and Name	*Specific Plants*	*Geographical Occurrence and Features*	*General Therapeutic Activity*
LABIATAE Lamiaceae	Lavender, Basil, Marjoram, Rosemary Thyme, Mint, Melissa, Patchouli, Hyssop	Temperate climatic zones, including Mediterranean and Britain.	Strong antiseptic, anti-spasmodic, digestive, vulnerary, bactericidal.
LAURACEAE	Rosewood, Cinnamon, Laurel, Litsea, Camphor	Mostly tropical and subtropical evergreen shrubs.	Cardiac stimulant, rubefacient, digestive, excretory, antiseptic, pulmonary.
MYRTACEAE divides into two subfamilies: Myrtoideae	Myrtle and Clove	Tropical and subtropical zones: Australia, East Indies and America.	Anti-fungal, anti-infectious, pectoral, expectorant, diuretic.
Leptospermoideae	Eucalyptus, Melaleuca family: Cajuput, Niaouli and Tea Tree		
PIPERACEAE	Black Pepper	Climbing plant that grows on trees in tropical monsoon regions. Grows in Malaysia, Southern India, South America and the West Indies.	Expectorant, anti-spasmodic, pectoral.
ROSACEAE	Rose Damask	Grows in temperate and subtropical climates in Europe, North Africa, Middle East and many other parts of the world.	Antitussive, anti-spasmodic, sedative, tonic.
RUTACEAE	Bergamot, Grapefruit, Lemon, Mandarin, Lime, Neroli, Orange, Petitgrain	Both temperate and tropical regions: Mediterranean region, Africa and South America.	Nervous tonic or sedatives, antiseptic, digestive, astringent, anti-scorbutic.

continued overleaf

Botanical Families *continued*			
Botanical Class and Name	Specific Plants	Geographical Occurrence and Features	General Therapeutic Activity
SANTALACEAE	Sandalwood	An evergreen tree, 8–12m tall and found mainly in southern India, East Indies and Australasia.	Diuretic, diaphoretic, expectorant, cooling and for genito-urinary system.
STYRACACEAE	Styrax Benzoin	Tropical trees and shrubs: Sumatra, Java, Malaysia and Indo-China.	Anti-inflammatory, astringent, expectorant, sedative.
UMBELLIFERAE Apiaceae	Angelica, Aniseed (*Pimpinella anethum*), Coriander, Fennel, Caraway, Carrot, Galbanum, Cumin	Found in temperate to tropical zones.	Excretory, digestive, anti-spasmodic, diuretic.
VERBANACEAE	Lemon Verbena	Temperate, tropical and subtropical zones.	Anti-spasmodic, digestive, nervous system tonic, neuromuscular, stomachic.
VIOLACEAE	Sweet Violet	Cold to temperate zones: northern hemisphere.	Expectorant, antitussive.
ZINGIBERACEAE	Ginger, Cardamon, Turmeric	Perennial aromatic herbs, growing in subtropical and tropical zones.	Stomachic, diaphoretic, prophylactic, carminative, circulatory stimulant.

CHAPTER 4
Chemical Classification of Essential Oils

THE NATURAL PRODUCTION OF ESSENTIAL OILS

The ecological sophistication of the world in which we live is a constant source of amazement to scientific observers, and with the new technology available for research and observation more and more is being discovered about the 'secret life of plants'.

What distinguishes an aromatic plant from other plants is the fact that it has a particular natural scent. People may not be aware of the difference between an aromatic plant and an ordinary plant, although in fact many aromatic plants are used every day as part of the food we consume – for example, herbs such as Basil, Thyme, Rosemary and Marjoram are all available fresh in many supermarkets. Their use in food reflects their properties that enhance the flavour of food and make it more digestible. I often point out to surprised students that essential oils are not synthetic, and that the art of extracting them from the plants is a scientific process which requires a certain knowledge.

Essential oils are not just any odd part of a plant, as they are the actual odorant chemicals which make up the particular smells of aromatic plants. There is no definitive answer as to why some plants have evolved to produce essential oils, but taking into account the nature of evolution, the fact that essential oils are produced at all means that they play some vital role in a plant's life cycle, be it for propagation and reproduction, for inflorescence (when in flower), or for healing the plant itself. Aromatic plants have fascinated many people throughout history, though none have seduced and inspired as much as the scented flora. Scented flowers are among the wonders of this world, attracting all sorts of creatures from insects, to birds, to human beings through their amazing smells. Essential oils can be found not just in flowers but also in the barks, roots and so on; their main purpose is to ensure the fertilization and reproduction of the plants.

Aromatic plants, like other plants, are entirely dependent upon symbiosis with their natural ecology. Their aromatic nature plays an intrinsic role in their survival. There are numerous essential oils, and each one has its own individual chemical signature and its own specific properties.

In each plant's own personal laboratory exists the mechanism by which a plant survives and grows – photosynthesis, the means by which plants convert water, CO_2, sunlight and nutrients into the building blocks necessary for growth, maintenance and propagation. The formation of essential oils is a miracle of biotechnology which occurs in the chloroplast deep within a plant's cells. Essential oils are the result of the multiple activities of chlorophyll macromolecules, whose vital task is to capture radiant energy from the sun. Essential oils are often a by-product of plant metabolism.

Within the plant cells there are also highly specialized secretory glands which likewise play a part in photosynthetic activities. It is specifically in these secretory cell glands that essential oils are produced and stored until climatic conditions or other factors force them out of their individual vesicles. In some plants the essential oils are stored just near the surface of the plant and can be observed without visual aid. This is the case with the skin of lemons or oranges where little dots can be seen and the essential oils can be forced out by squeezing the skin of the fruits.

Essential oils contain many chemical components which are the results of numerous transformations and evolutions while still in the plant. The diversity of the organic compounds found in the essential oils arises from carbon's unique ability to bond four times, allowing a near infinite number of molecular arrangements to take place. The chlorophyll units themselves are often cited as the 'factories' of the cell, where basic isoprene units join to form terpenes. A terpene is a structure that involves no other atoms than carbon (which forms the basic skeleton) and hydrogen. Due to the fact that the isoprene base unit has a five-carbon structure, all terpenic substances formed have carbon skeletons of either ten, fifteen or twenty atoms.

The progression to form further oxygenated constituents such as alcohols or phenols occurs as transformations to the initial terpenic units as a plant matures. Further transformations and reactions occur, reaching an equilibrium where hundreds of different chemicals are present, the 'blend' of which will give a plant essence its characteristics. The differences between the species lead to the variety of 'production paths' that are found in aromatic plants. It is these differences that give rise to the variety that exist in the constitutions of oils. For example, the path in *Cananga odorata* will be very different to that of *Eucalyptus globulus*.

There are a great many different types of aromatic plants, but not all of them yield enough essential oil to make the extraction process and expense worthwhile. Some of the oils can be highly toxic and therefore are not suitable for therapeutic purposes.

Depending upon the individual plant, essential oils can be found in the roots, bark, wood, branches, leaves, flowers, fruits and seeds. Different parts of a plant can produce different essential oils; for example, Angelica has three essential oils: one from its roots, one from its leaves and one from its seeds.

A part of the essential oils 'travels up' when the plant is ready to flower as they take part in reproduction. Alternatively, certain plants only produce essential oils in specific parts of their structure, as with Cinnamon or *Styrax benzoin* trees.

Characteristics of Essential Oils

Essential oils reveal a variety of physical and chemical characteristics. They can be: fluidic; odorant; coloured; volatile (although some of their chemicals evaporate quicker than others). They can undergo chemical changes when coming into contact with sunlight and air (oxygen and hydrogen and heat). They are not water soluble but will dissolve in pure alcohol, other chemical solvents or fatty oily substances. They are highly inflammable and must be kept at cool temperatures (around +5°C); and their density is usually lighter than water which often causes them to float on the surface (although some of them are heavier than water and sink to the bottom after distillation).

TABLES OF THE CHEMICAL CONSTITUENTS, MAIN THERAPEUTIC PROPERTIES AND POTENTIAL HAZARDS OF ESSENTIAL OILS

Monoterpenes			
Molecules have a ten-carbon atom base structure and a very faint odour.			
Examples	*Essential Oils Containing these Constituents*	*General Properties*	*Hazards and Toxicity*
Limonene	Lemon Orange Bergamot Pine	**All**: anti-viral, antiseptic, bactericidal, anti-inflammatory, diuretic, expectorant.	In quantities may cause skin and mucous membrane irritation if applied neat, according to the sensitivity of the skin. Symptoms may appear slowly and include redness, heat sensations and itchiness.
Pinene	Black Pepper Pine Angelica		
Camphene	Black Pepper		
Sylvestrene	Pine (Pine Sylvester)		
Dipentene	Lemon Grass Frankincense		
Myrcene	Bitter Orange		
Phelandrene	Fennel Clary Sage		
γ-Terpinene	Eucalyptus		
α-Sabinene	Black Pepper Juniper		

Sesquiterpenes			
Molecules are all based around a fifteen-carbon atom base structure and have a pleasant odour which is stronger than that of monoterpenes.			
Examples	*Essential Oils Containing these Constituents*	*General Properties*	*Hazards and Toxicity*
Camazulene	German Camomile	**All**: antiphlogistic, anti-inflammatory, cholagogue, antiseptic,	Can be toxic and may cause skin and mucous membrane irritation if applied neat, according to the sensitivity of the skin.
Viridifloral	Niaouli		

continued overleaf

Sesquiterpenes *continued*

Examples	*Essential Oils Containing these Constituents*	*General Properties*	*Hazards and Toxicity*
Cadinene	Cedarwood Ylang-Ylang	anti-epileptic, bactericidal, calming,	Symptoms may appear slowly and include redness, heat
Cedrene	Cedarwood	slight hypotensors, analgesic,	sensations and itchiness.
β-*Caryophyllene*	Clove Black Pepper Cedarwood	anti-carcinogenic.	

Sesquiterpinoids

Molecules are all based around a fifteen-carbon atom base structure with an additional functional group. This interaction between the carbonic chain and the functional group is very subtle.

Examples	*Essential Oils Containing these Constituents*	*General Properties*	*Hazards and Toxicity*
Bisabolol alcohol	German Camomile	**All**: anti-phlogistic, disinfectant,	Can be toxic and may cause skin and mucous membrane irritation if
α-*Santalol alcohol*	Sandalwood	antiseptic, bacteriostatic, deodorizing,	applied neat, according to the sensitivity of the skin. Symptoms may
Farnesol alcohol	Rose Roman Camomile	dermatophillic, stomachic, carminative.	appear slowly and include redness, heat sensations and
Zingiberol alcohol	Ginger	**Some are**: analgesic, spasmolytic.	itchiness.

Diterpenes

Molecules are all based around a twenty-carbon atom base structure and have very little odour.

Examples	*Essential Oils Containing these Constituents*	*General Properties*	*Hazards and Toxicity*
α-*Camphorene*	Camphor	**All**: antiseptic bactericidal, expectorant, purgative.	As above in quantities and depending on sensitivity of skin can be toxic.

Examples	Essential Oils Containing these Constituents	General Properties	Hazards and Toxicity
		Some: have a balancing effect on the hormonal system, are anti-fungal, anti-viral, anti-carcinogenic.	

Diterpinoids

Molecules are all based around a twenty-carbon atom structure with an additional functional group. This interaction between the carbonic chain and the functional group is very subtle.

Examples	Essential Oils Containing these Constituents	General Properties	Hazards and Toxicity
Sclareol (*alcohol*)	Clary Sage	**All**: antiseptic, bactericidal, expectorant, purgative. **Some**: have a balancing effect on the hormonal system, are anti-fungal, anti-viral, anti-carcinogenic.	Can be toxic.

Aldehydes

The properties of this particular carbonyl group operate halfway between alcohols and ketones. They are found in essential oils with a lemon scent (citral) and have a powerful and often 'fruity' aroma.

Functional group, suffix -al

Examples	Essential Oils Containing these Constituents	General Properties	Hazards and Toxicity
Citral (the name given to the 'mixture' of its two stereoisomers, Neral and Geranial).	Melissa Lemon Grass Citronella	Sedative, yet uplifting, aldehydes tend to be anti-inflammatory and relaxants of the nervous system (vasodilator and hypotensor).	Non toxic. Aldehydes may cause skin irritation and sensitivity if used incorrectly.

continued overleaf

Aldehydes *continued*

Examples	*Essential Oils Containing these Constituents*	*General Properties*	*Hazards and Toxicity*
Citronellal	Lemon Verbena Eucalyptus Mandarin	They are antiseptic (citral being especially strong) and anti-viral.	They may also irritate mucous membranes.
Benzaldehyde	Cinnamon		
Cinnamic aldehyde	Cinnamon		

Ketones

Both ketones and aldehydes contain the carbonyl functional group, C=O, making them structurally similar. The difference in where the carbonyl group is placed within the molecule gives us the considerable difference in properties. The carbonyl group in aldehydes is placed at the end of the chain, whereas in ketones it is placed within the chain.

$$-C-C-C-$$ Functional group, suffix -one

Examples	*Essential Oils Containing these Constituents*	*General Properties*	*Hazards and Toxicity*
Thuyone	Hyssop	**All:** Cicatrisant, cyto-phylactic, lipolytic, mucolytic, sedative, promotes the healing of scar tissue, can get rid of certain parasites such as worms and mycosis and are also a powerful respiratory decongestant. Some of the ketones such as those found in Hyssop (Thuyone) have remarkable properties reputed to treat success-fully chronic respiratory complaints, particularly when mucus is blocking/congesting this system. Some ketones are anti-coagulant, anti-inflam-matory, digestive, analgesic and immune stimulants.	Although not all ketones are dangerous, internal absorption can cause abortion, convulsion, epilepsy, stupor and sometimes even death. The prolonged use of oils with a high ketone content is not recommended as it could cause neuro-toxicity, hepato-toxicity and kidney damage.
Pinocamphone	Hyssop		
Carvone	Peppermint		
Jasmone	Jasmine Neroli		
Fenchone	Sweet Fennel Basil Marjoram		
Camphone	Peppermint		
Menthone	Peppermint Thyme		

Terpenic Alcohols			
Terpenic alcohols have a terpene base structure with a hydroxyl group attached to one of the carbons and are the first oxygenated compounds to be formed in the synthesis of essential oils. They have pleasant, uplifting fragrances.			

$-\mathrm{C-O-H}$ Functional group, suffix -ol

Examples	*Essential Oils Containing these Constituents*	*General Properties*	*Hazards and Toxicity*
Linalol	Lavender Rosewood Petitgrain Coriander Neroli	They are far less aggressive than the phenols, and can be safely used on children. **All:** stimulating,	Very low toxicity. Do not cause skin irritation.
Borneol	Sandalwood	antiseptic, positively energizing, tonic for	
Citronellol	Rose Lemon Geranium Eucalyptus	the nervous system, strongly bactericidal, anti-fungal, antibiotic, immune response stimulant, vaso-	
Geraniol	Geranium Palmarosa	constrictors. **Citronellol**: anti-viral.	
α-Santalol *β-Santalol*	Sandalwood		
α-Terpineol	Niaouli Eucalyptus		
Terpineol-4	Tea Tree Garden Marjoram Juniper		
Myrtenol	Myrtle		
Vetiverol	Vetivert		
Nerol	Neroli		
Farnesol	Palmarosa		
Menthol	Peppermint		
Cedrol	Cedarwood		

Phenols

Although aliphatic (non-cyclic) alcohols and phenols both contain the hydroxyl group, (-O-H), their strength and properties are considerably different. The phenol molecule itself was used by Dr Joseph Lister in the 1860s as one of the first antiseptics in surgery and the antiseptic and anti-infectious properties of phenolic compounds are unsurpassed even in modern pharmacology.

Functional group and the phenol molecule itself, suffix -ol

Examples	Essential Oils Containing these Constituents	General Properties	Hazards and Toxicity
Thymol	Thyme	**All:** anti-bacterial agents, (carvacrol and thymol are especially strong), antiseptic, immunostimulant, stimulant for central nervous system, tend to increase heat in the body. **Eugenol:** fungicidal, local anaesthetic, inhibits certain carcinogenic functions. **Carvacrol:** a highly toxic phenol, has great anti-infectious properties. These oils could trigger convulsions or even epileptic fits in people who are prone to them.	**VERY HAZARDOUS** Essential oils with a high content of phenols should be used in smaller quantities, well diluted in vegetable oils and the therapist should pay attention to the nervous state of the client/patient before use. They should not be used neat or over a long period of time. In larger doses, they become a powerful excitant and poison to the nervous system and are powerful skin irritants. They are also hepatoxic (toxic to the liver).
Carvacrol	Thyme		
Eugenol	Cinnamon Clove		

Esters

Esters are formed by a condensation reaction between a carboxylic acid and an alcohol which bond across an oxygen by eliminating water. They are known for their sweet-smelling, fruity odours are the most commonly found group of the essential oil constituents.

Functional group, alcohol + suffix -yl, then acid + suffix -ate

Examples	Essential Oils Containing these Constituents	General Properties	Hazards and Toxicity
Linalyl acetate	Lavender Bergamot Clary Sage	**All:** Especially efficient in rebalancing and relaxing the nervous system, esters are anti-spasmodic, anti-inflammatory, anti-fungal, sedative, spasmolytic (especially Roman Camomile), calming to the central nervous system, cicatrisant, anti-bacterial, very gentle on the skin.	In therapeutic doses, there are no known toxicities – 'user friendly'.
Geranyl acetate	Sweet Marjoram Petitgrain		
Bornyl acetate	Pine Rosemary		
Methyl acetate	Peppermint		
Eugenyl acetate	Cinnamon Leaf		
Lavendulyl acetate	Lavender		
Benzyl acetate	Jasmine Ylang-Ylang		
Methyl salicylate	Ylang-Ylang		
Methyl benzoate	Ylang-Ylang		
Cinnamyl acetate	Cinnamon		
Myrtinyl acetate	Myrtle		

33

Oxides

The oxygen itself forms part of the ring structural base unit. Oxides are found in small quantities in most essential oils.

Examples	Essential Oils Containing these Constituents	General Properties	Hazards and Toxicity
Cineol (also known as Eucalyptol)	Eucalyptus Rosemary Tea Tree and found as a small proportion in almost every other essential oil	**All:** expectorant, mucolytic, glandular stimulants. Linalol oxide is excellent for asthma as it has a mild anti-inflammatory action and is mucolytic. Oxides also show eupeptic, stomachic and carminative properties.	Oxides tend to be strong skin irritants, especially to young children. Used in quantity or over a long period of time, oxides can be neuro-toxic.
Linalol oxide	Hyssop		
Bisabolol oxide	German Camomile		
Bisabolone oxide	German Camomile		
Piperitone oxide	Black Pepper		

Coumarins

Coumarins are otherwise known as heterocyclic lactones. Coumarin itself has an odour of freshly mown hay.

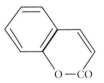

Functional group and coumarin itself. Suffixes -in and -ene.

Examples	Essential Oils Containing these Constituents	General Properties	Hazards and Toxicity
Coumarin	Grapefruit Lime	Coumarins tend to act on the circulatory system (especially the blood) and the nervous system.	Coumarins are highly photosensitive and oils containing citroptene or beroptene should be used carefully (found mostly in citruses), coumarins have low volatility, and tend
Archangelicin (also known as angelicin)	Angelica		

Examples	Essential Oils Containing these Constituents	General Properties	Hazards and Toxicity
Imperatonin Citroptene	Angelica Found in all citruses	**All:** anti-coagulants, hypotensors, thought to be anti-convulsives, uplifting yet sedative (reduce the degree of hyperactivity of reflexes).	to act on the skin for longer than the other components. This becomes especially hazardous when people are exposed to the sun many hours after a treatment, as the oils can still cause tissue damage to the underlying layers of the skin. Essential oils in dilution can remain active up to 70 hours after application. For hyper-sensitive skins, lactones can cause skin and mucous membrane allergies. The pyran-coumarins are hepato-toxic.

Furanocoumarins

Occur particularly in *Rutaceae* and *Umbelliferae*.

Examples	Essential Oils Containing these Constituents	General Properties	Hazards and Toxicity
Bergapten	Bergamot Sweet Orange Grapefruit	Anti-viral, anti-fungal.	The furanocoumarins tend to become photo-sensitizers when they come into contact with the sun. Essential oils in dilution will remain active for up to 70 hours after application.

Lactones			
Lactones are organic cyclic esters where the ester group forms part of a ring structure. Lactones are not so commonly found in essential oils.			

Functional group, suffix -lactone.

Examples	Essential Oils Containing these Constituents	General Properties	Hazards and Toxicity
Santalactone	Sandalwood	**All:** mucolytic,	Can cause dermatitis. If taken orally, they
g-undecalactone (odour of peaches)	Sandalwood	expectorant, febrifuge.	become neuro-toxic and can have similar negative effects to ketones. They
g-nonalactone (odour of coconut)	Sandalwood		also have a sensitizing effect on the skin and increase phototoxicity.

PROCESS OF EXTRACTION OF ESSENTIAL OILS

Earthlier happy is the rose distill'd
Than that which withers on the virgin thorn.
William Shakespeare

The separation of essential oils from their plants is a very delicate procedure, and the choice of method to achieve this is determined by their intended use later on. The cosmetic, pharmacy and food industries all make great use of essential oils; comparatively, the Aromatherapy profession only accounts for a small fraction of the total essential oil production. The art of extracting essential oils by means of water or steam distillation is fairly ancient, but it was not until the 1800s that a reliable instrument was available to produce finer quality. Over the centuries, the methods of extraction have steadily improved, and some of the extraction procedures today are very sophisticated and effective.

The still was invented around the 11th Century by Avicenna, a famous Persian philosopher and doctor nicknamed the 'king of doctors' (980–1037), who also wrote the *Cannon of Medicine*, a treatise taught to medical students right up to the end of the 17th Century. Holy Crusaders who travelled to the Orient brought back to Europe great inventions and new skills. From the 11th Century onwards, physicians, philosophers and alchemists became obsessed with the secret of immortality. Turning lead into gold would be proof that they had achieved the transmutation of cosmic energies and transcended the dimension of the physical world. The alembic, a flask or vessel used for the distillation of plants' essences, was an important instrument in alchemy and its purpose was to distil 'the spirit' or 'quintessence' of the plants and use this elixir for spiritual transformation. The alembic was a symbol of purification. Another famous philosopher, physician and surgeon, Paracelsus, whose real name was Phillipus Aureolus Bombastus Von Honeheim (16th Century) and who was also a fervent alchemist, succeeded in separating the gross part of plants from their more subtle components, isolating certain chemical substances to make new reme-dies. He was credited with naming the 'quintessences' of plants 'essential oils'. It was also during this period that distillation began to become more precise and deliver purer essential oils, although mostly in small quantities.

Around the 15th Century, the Germans and a few Italians had become masters at the art of distillation of essential oils for use in perfumery and medicinal remedies.

In 1826, Beindorff, a German engineer, invented an instrument of distillation at 'low pressure' suitable for pharmacists. This man's invention was so well designed and gave such satisfactory results that it became the standard model to much of the still apparatus available today all over the world.

The Modern Production of Essential Oils

Modern stills are built to ensure that the natural odour of plants and the fine balance between the many individual chemical constituents are not submitted to any significant changes while undergoing distillation. In theory, extraction by distillation sounds simple, but in reality the quality of essential oils is down to the type of apparatus used and the knowledge of the supervising chemist and his experience of distilling a particular plant. For example, Lavender has different distillation requirements to Geranium. When I go to the French Provence at the time of the distillation of Lavender, I drive around the distilleries, which are usually situated in very remote places in the mountains. There, it is amusing to see how people who distil the oil treat it with the same love and pride as the nearby wine producers treat their vintage wines. The quality of the essential oils is a vital factor in Aromatherapy, as it determines the therapeutic capacity of each essential oil. In all cases, 'purest is best'.

There are a number of other methods of extraction apart from distillation, but the products from some of them are not suitable for use in Aromatherapy.

Each industry which uses essential oils has different criteria in terms of the quality. For example, the food industry is more concerned about preserving the odour/flavour of the essential oils than maintaining the fine balance of the chemical components, so long as the final product is safe. The pharmaceutical industry, on the other hand, is more concerned about isolating the individual chemical agents in order to combine them with other types of components in medicinal remedies. The cosmetics industry is only concerned with the chemical components as a means to recognize and label which ingredients are going into a product or how to reproduce the fragrance. In Aromatherapy, the 'whole' essential oil in its purest form is used to achieve an overall therapeutic effect. This is because the human body appears to tolerate natural substances a lot better than synthetic pharmacy; they also tend to encourage the body's defence system to do its own healing. Aromatherapists also seek to heal by stimulating the sense of smell in order to achieve an altered state of mind which may bring into play unconscious processes that can restore harmony and balance.

As a result of these differences in purpose there has been some debate among Aromatherapists and pharmacists regarding the validity of using the totality of an essential oil or only its most active agents. Many authorities in the field hold the view that it is more efficient and safer for the body to use the whole essential oil, as certain components tend to counterbalance others. Some chemical constituents are only found in minute quantities while others are found in abundance, and it is this factor that gives each essential oil its therapeutic capacity. The only drawback is that when the 'whole' essential oil is used it is difficult to establish which particular chemical component actually acts upon a symptom or ailment. However, in this debate, safety is the paramount consideration while treating patients, and therefore if an essential oil does represent a danger to health its use should be prohibited altogether. Here it is appropriate to quote the old saying 'if in doubt, abstain'.

Finally, to reflect the complex nature of essential oils, here is the technical description of essential oils as written down by the Essential Oil Technical Committee of the International Standards Organisation: 'The odoriferous products obtained by steam distillation of plant material from a specific botanical source or by expression of the pericarp of citrus fruits and their separation by physical methods from the aqueous phase.'

ANCIENT AND MODERN METHODS OF EXTRACTING ESSENTIAL OILS FROM PLANTS

Perfumes are the feeling of flowers.
Heinrich Heine

Expression

This method is used for the extraction of essential oils from citrus fruits, such as Bergamots, Mandarins, Lemons, Oranges, Grapefruits and Limes and they are particularly in demand by the food industry as they are used to flavour food. Only the rind of the fruit contains essential oils and the rest of the fruit is disregarded.

Expression involves moistening the skin of the fruit and manually scratching or grating it to puncture the vesicles where essential oils are stored; constant use of water spray on the fruit collects the oil. Today, industrial methods have replaced traditional manual ones and the fruit rind is lacerated with metal spikes and squeezed by machines. Both juice and essence are collected together then separated later. This is much faster than the earlier method

but the essential oil is not necessarily as fine. The essential oils produced by this method are the closest chemically to the essential oils found in plants. The difference between expression and distillation is that the latter requires water and heat and these can destroy some of the more volatile chemical components and alter the exact chemical composition of essential oil constituents. Some of the other methods described below are used by the perfume and cosmetic industries and can produce certain residues, such as animal and vegetable oils, petroleum ethers and so on, and are not necessarily suitable for use in Aromatherapy.

Distillation

Until the 18th Century essential oils were not freely available in the market place as the methods used to extract them were not able to produce quantities. Sometimes the oils were not as pure as they would be today either, which made them difficult to use.

18th-Century Distillation in France

The collection and distillation of wild aromatic plants in Haute Provence in the 19th Century, required the travelling merchants to go to the fields high up on the side of the mountains and to camp out for the duration of the distillation period. The stills with their cooling coils and steam chambers were transported by carts or on the backs of mules to a makeshift camp by a clear-water spring (as good water is important to distillation). The plants were gathered up and collected in large bundles and carried back to the camp, and for most plants the cuttings had to be processed while they were still fresh. The merchants kept on moving on, repeating this operation until they had obtained enough essential oils and were ready to take them down to the various specialized small town markets, such as Montbrun-les-bains, for sale where they would get a good price for them. This is still practised in places like Morocco and other developing countries.

Modern-Day Distillation

Distillation apparatuses can be simple or very complex depending on the plants to be distilled and the country where it takes place. There are two types of distillation: one is water distillation and the other is steam distillation. Some plants require both. For steam distillation, low pressure distillation is more suitable for much of the production of essential oils used in Aromatherapy. This is because many of the chemicals in essential oils are highly volatile and get easily destroyed by the heat, and too much heat will 'lift' other thicker materials such as gums. The coarser parts of plants make essential oils less pure and less therapeutically active. Distillation at high pressure is more likely to be used in the cosmetic and perfumery industries where therapeutics is not the aim. Both require the supervision of an expert chemist to get the best results. The use of pesticides and modern fertilizers on crops also creates a problem regarding the purity of essential oils, so whenever possible organically grown or wild plants are preferable to chemically fertilized cultivated aromatic plants.

Description of a Still and the Distillation Process

This method is mainly used for flowers, stems, leaves, seeds, fruits, barks, some resins, wood and roots. Flowers, leaves and stems do not require any special preparation but aromatic material such as wood or bark may need to be dried, heated or broken down before distillation can take place.

Water Distillation

With water distillation the plants are immersed in water and heated externally by fire or electrical means. This is the simplest and cheapest method and is very frequently used in developing countries, but it has drawbacks: it is labour intensive and time consuming and the actual smell of the flowers can be spoiled easily. However, certain plant material can only be distilled with this method, as is the case with Rose petals or Orange blossoms.

Instruments of distillation can be described as a collection of sealed metal containers that can resist pressure and heat.

Water/Steam Distillation

This is the most common form of distillation and is much quicker than the former one as the heat is greater. However, it can only be used for aromatic material.

The first container is used to heat up water and produce steam; the steam travels through a tube to the next vessel which contains the aromatic material. The plants in the second vessel are usually laid on a suspended perforated tray and as the steam passes through, it releases the volatile essential oils. The essential oils then travel up as part of the steam to the next container. This third container is fitted inside with a 'serpentine' (a coiled tube) and immersed in cold water. As the aromatic vapours rush through the coil, the cold water acts as a cooling agent and condenses the essential oils back to their liquid form. They are then collected and separated from the water and sold separately.

'Rectification' is a procedure used when it is necessary to improve the essential oil for a particular reason, often to remove unwanted terpenes; it is usually done with fractional distillation. Distilled waters, such as rose water, are a by-product of essential oils' distillation and are also called 'hydrolats'. Interestingly, most distillation instruments evolved because of the great demand over the centuries for distilled waters while the demand for essential oils was less common and the market for them much smaller. This is not the case today.

Fragrant Material Extraction with Fixed Solvents, Hexane or Petroleum Spirit

Enfleurage: fixed solvent extraction

This method is the oldest perfumery method and is quite rare nowadays as it is time consuming and little oil can be produced in this way; it is also very expensive to produce. It requires panes of glass mounted on rectangular wooden frames (called chassis), animal or vegetable fat and flower petals. The fat is painted on the glass surface and the frame is filled up with flower petals, usually petals from the more delicate flowers such as Violet or Jasmine. Several frames are treated in this manner at the same time and when they are ready, they are stacked up upon each other and left to distil naturally in the heat of the sun. This procedure is repeated every day or every few days depending on what type of flowers are being processed at the time. This will go on for several weeks until the 'fixe' oil is saturated with essential oil. The fat is then collected and, at this stage, it is known as 'pomade for washing'. The fat is then dissolved in ethanol to separate essential oils from it, the ethanol will be evaporated from the essential oil through a delicate procedure at a later time.

Sometimes, instead of 'chassis' and the heat of the sun, the aromatic plants are immersed in the 'fixe' oil, usually vegetable oil, and heated up to facilitate the release of aromas. This is then called maceration.

Fragrance Material Extraction by Maceration

This process is mostly used for cosmetic and perfumery ends and involves aromatic materials and the 'fixe' oil being placed together in large vessels which are heated up to about 65–70°C. The heat and regular stirring help the release of essential oils in the 'fixe' oil. When the maceration is deemed sufficient, the containers are emptied on a net placed on a large perforated tray and left to drain. Further quantities of flowers will be added to the oil until it is saturated. The net is later spun in a centrifuge to collect the last of the oil.

Fragrance Material Extraction by Volatile Solvents

This method is very much in use today particularly for the collection of the natural fragrance of the more delicate flowers such as: Jasmine, Rose, Carnation, Violet, Mimosa and Narcissus, all of which contain only minute quantities of essential oils in their flowers.

The most common method involves the use of petroleum and, of course, flower petals. The aromatic material is sprayed with the solvent and left to stand for some hours to allow the solvent to be absorbed by the flowers and to force the release of the essential oil from the petals. The solvent is then recovered under vacuum and, at this stage, part of the by-product of the distillation is semi-solid as much of the natural waxes from the flowers have also been released. One more procedure is now needed to restore the fluidity of the oil as the waxes need to be removed and pure alcohol is used for this particularly delicate operation. The whole operation has to be carefully executed to reproduce exactly the scent of the flower. The essential oil obtained through this method will still contain traces of solvent and is only helpful in Aromatherapy when using essential oils for the psychological therapeutic benefits of their scents and not for the other therapeutic effects essential oils may have on the human body. The essential oils obtained in this manner are also known as flora absolutes and should certainly never be taken internally.

Essential Oil General Chart Data				
Names	*Latin Names*	*Botanical Family*	*Part of Plant the Oil is Obtained from*	*Method of Extraction*
Angelica Root	*Angelica archangelica*	Umbelliferae/ Apiaceae	Root	Distillation
Star Aniseed	*Illicium verum*	Illiciaceae	Fruit	Distillation
Basil (Sweet)	*Occimum basilicum*	Labiatae/ Lamiaceae	Leaves	Distillation
Benzoin	*Styrax benzoin*	Styraceae	Resin	Solvent extraction
Bergamot	*Citrus aurantium* var. *bergamia*	Rutaceae	Rind	Expression
Black Pepper	*Piper nigrun*	Piperaceae	Fruit	Distillation
Camomile (German)	*Matricaria chamomilla, M. recutita*	Compositae/ Asteraceae	Flowers	Distillation
Camomile (Roman)	*Anthemis nobilis, Chamaemelum nobile*	Compositae/ Asteraceae	Flowers	Distillation
Cedarwood	*Cedrus atlantica*	Coniferae	Wood	Distillation
Cinnamon	*Cinnamomum verum, C. zeylanicum*	Lauraceae	Leaf	Distillation
Clary Sage	*Salvia sclarea*	Labiatae/ Lamiaceae	Aerial Parts	Distillation

continued overleaf

Essential Oil General Chart Data *continued*				
Names	*Latin Names*	*Botanical Family*	*Part of Plant the Oil is Obtained from*	*Method of Extraction*
Coriander	*Coriandrum sativum*	Umbelliferae/ Apiaceae	Seeds/Leaves	Distillation
Cypress	*Cupressus* var. *stricta, Cupressus sempervirens*	Coniferae var. Cupressaceae	Leaves/New Stems	Distillation
Eucalyptus	*Eucalyptus globulus, Eucalyptus citriodora*	Myrtaceae	Leaves	Distillation
Fennel (sweet)	*Foeniculum vulgare* var. *dulce*	Umbelliferae/ Apiaceae	Seeds	Distillation
Frankincense	*Boswellia corterii, Boswellia thurifera*	Burseraceae	Resin	Distillation
Geranium	*Pelargonium odorantissimum, Graveolens*	Geraniaceae	Aerial Parts	Distillation
Ginger	*Zingiber officinale*	Zingiberaceae	Rhizome	Distillation
Grapefruit	*Citrus grandisi, Martinii* or *Citrus* var. *paradisii*	Rutaceae	Rind	Expression
Jasmine (Abs)	*Jasmine grandiflorum*	Jasminaceae	Flowers	Solvent extraction
Juniper Berry	*Juniperus communis* ssp. *communis* var. *juniperus*	Coniferae var. Cupressaceae	Berries	Distillation
Lavender	*Lavendula officinalis, L. angustifolia*	Labiatae/Lamiaceae	Flowering Tops	Distillation

Names	Latin Names	Botanical Family	Part of Plant the Oil is Obtained from	Method of Extraction
Lemon	*Citrus limon*	Rutaceae	Rind	Expression
Lemon Grass	*Cymbopogon citratus*	Gramineae	Aerial Parts	Distillation
Lime	*Citrus aurantifolia*	Rutaceae	Rind	Expression
Mandarin	*Citrus reticulata madurensis*	Rutaceae	Rind	Expression
Marjoram	*Origanum marjorana*	Labiatae/Lamiaceae	Flowering Tops/Leaf	Distillation
Melissa	*Melissa officinalis*	Labiatae/Lamiaceae	Stems/Leaf	Distillation
Myrrh	*Commiphora abyssinica, Myrrha mollmol, Commiphora mollmol*	Burseraceae	Gum/Resin	Distillation
Myrtle	*Myrtus communis*	Myrtaceae	Stems/Leaf	Distillation
Neroli	*Citrus aurantium* var. *amara*	Rutaceae	Flowers	Distillation
Niaouli	*Melaleuca quinquinerva, M. veridiflora*	Myrtaceae	Leaf	Distillation
Orange (Bitter)	*Citrus aurantium* × *amaroi*	Rutaceae	Rind	Expression
Orange (Sweet)	*Citrus aurantium* × *sinensis*	Rutaceae	Rind	Expression
Palmarosa	*Cymbopogon martinii*	Gramineae	Aerial Parts	Distillation
Patchouli	*Pogostemon patchouli*	Labiatae/Lamiaceae	Aerial Parts	Distillation

continued overleaf

Essential Oil General Chart Data *continued*				
Names	*Latin Names*	*Botanical Family*	*Part of Plant the Oil is Obtained from*	*Method of Extraction*
Peppermint	*Mentha piperita*	Labiatae/Lamiaceae	Leaves	Distillation
Petitgrain	*Citrus aurantium*	Rutaceae	Stems	Distillation
Pine	*Pinus sylvestris*	Coniferae/Apiaceae	Needles	Distillation
Rose	*Rosa damascena, R. centifolia (Otto)*	Rosaceae	Petals	Distillation
Rose (Abs)	*Rosa damascena*	Rosaceae	Petals/ Rose Leaves	Solvent extraction
Rosemary	*Rosmarinus officinalis*	Labiatae/Lamiaceae	Flowering Tops, Leaves	Distillation
Rosewood	*Aniba rosaeodora*	Lauraceae	Leaf	Distillation
Sandalwood	*Santalum album*	Myrtaceae	Stems/Leaves	Distillation
Tea Tree	*Melaleuca alternifolia*	Myrtaceae	Stems/Leaves	Distillation
Thyme	*Thymus vulgaris*	Labiatae/Lamiaceae	Flowering Stems and Tops	Distillation
Verbena (Lemon)	*Lippia citriodora*	Verbenaceae	Leaf	Distillation
Vetivert	*Vetiveria zizanoides*	Gramineae	Root	Distillation
Violet (Abs)	*Viola odorata*	Violaceae	Leaves	Solvent extraction
Ylang-Ylang	*Cananga odorata*	Annonaceae	Flowers	Distillation

CHAPTER 5
The Art of Healing with Scents

The sense of smell is especially effective in arousing memories.
Nothing awakens a reminiscence like an odour.
Schopenhauer

THE ART OF THE PERFUMER

Perfumery is the art of combining diverse scented material to create a 'perfume' that will stimulate the sense of smell and generate sensory reactions throughout our being.

The sensations that perfumes produce can be physical or subtle, and can also be very revitalizing. Different scents or perfumes can be experienced as soothing, comforting or simply steal our senses away.

Literature about perfumes is often deeply eloquent. Perfumers are truly wizards in disguise and masters of illusions who expertly manipulate our senses with enchanted vapours. They initiate scented harmonies and playfully awaken long-lost memories of adventure or romance in faraway places, leading us on a scented tour of the inner temple where the smoke of burning Frankincense endlessly rises towards a forfeited Paradise. Incense is said to be the ancestor of perfumes and has been burnt over the centuries for many reasons, often being used as an intercessor between humans and Gods.

There are also special scents for special occasions – Rose is the Queen of Hearts, Jasmine brings lovers to the courtesan, Verbena revives the love of life, Myrrh induces an urge for penance and purification and Frankincense will uplift the soul.

Creating Healing Perfumes

Creating a harmonious blend of essential oils for a treatment that requires physiological and psychological benefits is always going to be a challenge. To accomplish this task Aromatherapists have to acquire methodology and skills combined with a certain 'know how', all of which can only be gained through training and repeated practice.

The psycho-physiological effect of essential oils when applied correctly can help redress the loss of equilibrium between mind and body, as it can encourage proper healing from deep in the mind. The biggest psychological factor currently responsible for many illnesses in modern society is stress, which can be mental or physical or both. Many psychosomatic ailments can be difficult to rectify because of their psychological origins. Relaxation ought to play a vital role in the treatment of such diseases, coupled with the appropriate medicinal remedy.

In fact, stress is not necessarily the cause of illness, but rather the impelling force behind the development of existing minor problems.

For example, if physical tiredness or an emotional crisis 'stresses someone out', physical symptoms will become more acute, therefore creating even more stress. In time, a vicious circle of stress/increasing symptoms will be created, which may lead to permanent damage to the body.

To address physical and psychological 'hurt', the Aromatherapist has to learn to manage a two-sided approach, that is, a treatment which will alleviate physical symptoms as well as ease mental suffering. Physiological problems that create discomfort must be the first thing to take into account when assessing the correct choice of treatment. The therapeutic benefits derived from the external application of essential oils are dealt with in Chapters 6 and 7.

The second factor that determines the choice of treatment relates more to moods, the state of mind and feelings. The psychological benefits that essential oils can provide for this complex aspect of human life occur as a result of sensory stimulation when our sense of smell encounters any scented molecules. It is a known scientific fact that the sense of smell has a direct connection to the brain. The Aromatherapist's first step to therapeutic blending, therefore, is to learn how to recognize the many components of essential oils, assess their strength and sensory effects and blend them in a harmonious manner.

All Aromatherapists need to acquire some of the skills of the perfumer and some of the skills of the physician; knowledge of both can help to achieve a more holistic treatment. It is not easy to work with the concentrated essences from plants and the secret of blending is to play with the different components of a smell until they have formed a harmonious melody. Most of us will have experienced smells which were so repellent that they made us cringe with disgust; the Aromatherapist is aiming for the opposite effect, which will lead to a 'cure' for the mind as well as the body.

Three Steps to Harmonious Blending

1. The first step towards learning to create a therapeutic and harmonious blend is to become fluent in the general therapeutic properties of essential oils.
2. The second step is to acquire an understanding of the olfactory system and the general effects that scents have on the central nervous system. The way people are affected by smells and more particularly essential oils can vary. The effects may be psychological, such as altering moods, or a physiological reaction may be triggered.
3. Thirdly, an experiential study of the traditional approach to the art of perfume making will lead to a better ability to choose scents and create a 'harmonious' blend. The practical experience of smelling a great variety of scents helps to develop an awareness of the various components in a smell. To expand the faculty of olfactory discrimination it is necessary to gain a wider vocabulary of terms referring to the description of smells.

OLFACTORY SCIENCE

The experience of odour and the experience of emotion are, in some basic physiological way, the same. Molecules of odour seem to stimulate the brain centres that signal the basic drives underlying all human emotion.

Dr Howard Ehrlichman, City University of New York

What is the Sense of Smell?

The sense of smell is one of the five senses that allow us to interpret the external world. Generally, sense perception is triggered by an external factor and its purpose is to analyse this factor, define its qualities and make connections if possible. Each of our senses is activated into analytic mode when it comes into contact with its particular element, for example: hearing is activated by sound; seeing by light; smelling by odour; taste by flavour; and touch by coming into contact with a range of sensations. Very often, what is thought of as a flavour in food turns out to be a smell and vice versa as the two are often confused.

What is Olfaction?

This is the sensory process which responds to odorant chemical stimuli (odours) and gives rise to olfactory sensations (stimuli). This neural process permits communication between the outside world, our olfactory receptors and our brain.

What are Smell Sensations?

Smell sensations are caused by airborne molecules entering the nose and meeting with olfactory receptors. The molecules get caught on the membrane fluid where they dissolve and interact with the ciliate membrane, and it is this interaction between the two that gives rise to odour sensations. Odorant chemicals need to be volatile (that is, in a gaseous state) to travel with the air to olfactory receptors in the nose. They also need to be both fat-soluble and small enough to diffuse through the epithelial membrane and react with the olfactory receptors. When the sensations occur they are then relayed to the brain for analysis and response.

What is the Purpose of Olfaction?

Olfaction seems to have developed to protect us from possible external dangers such as predators and also to enable us to find food. It helps us to identify aspects of the environment in which we live, as we need to find food, recognize dangers, or even select potential sexual partners for reproduction.

It is generally an accepted fact that in terms of research the scientific study of the sense of smell has lagged behind that of the other senses, yet experts in the field regard the sense of smell as being 'the window to the brain' because of its direct connection to it.

Anatomical Description of the Sense of Smell

Key terms:
Olfactory system
Olfactory epithelium
Olfactory receptor cells
Olfactory nerve
Olfactory bulb
Olfactory cortex

Olfactory Epithelium

The olfactory epithelium is found on each side of the upper part of the nasal septum. This area is also called the olfactory cleft. The olfactory epithelium is made up of three layers of membranes containing basal cells, supporting cells and olfactory receptor cells.

What are Olfactory Receptor Cells?

Olfactory receptor cells are sensory neurones that respond to odorant chemicals, many of them reacting to very specific chemicals. We possess anything between 10–100,000 million olfactory receptor cells. Specialized areas of olfactory neurones tend to respond to 'primary' smells. Some of the most common detectable smells are believed to be a combination of a small range of smells, about fifty in number.

Odorant chemicals are not carried in the inner membranes as such, but, rather, trigger a modified reaction when in contact with cells.

47

Location of Olfactory Receptors

Olfactory neurones are part of the olfactory mucosa, that lies on the central part of the ethmoid bone and is a continuation of the nasal septum higher up. Each receptor cell has an extended projection called the axon, through which sensory information (smells) are transmitted to the olfactory bulb. The dendrites of olfactory neurones extend to the nasal cavities and form a bulbous enlargement called olfactory vesicles. These have very fine hair-like olfactory cilia (microvilli) and are coated with a fluidic film which collects odour molecules. The cilia are also called 'olfactory hair'. The olfactory tract extends from the olfactory bulb and joins with the olfactory cortex in the brain.

Description of the Olfactory Nerve

The olfactory nerve is the first of the cranial nerves. It is the extension of the cells which form the olfactory mucosa in the nasal cavity. The axons of the olfactory neurones project through the cribriform plate of the ethmoid bone and end in the olfactory bulbs.

The Function of the Olfactory Bulbs

The olfactory bulbs are the primary centre for the transmission of olfactory information to the brain; they are also the most direct contact our brain has with its immediate environment. Messages, which enter the olfactory bulbs, are analysed and sent to the olfactory cortex for response.

Olfactory Dysfunction

- **Anosmia**: inability to detect odour sensations; absence of sense of smell.
- **Hyposmia**: decreased sensitivity to some or all odours (smokers are often said to have a lowered sense of smell).
- **Hyperosmia**: increased sensitivity to some or all odours; often occurs during pregnancy.
- **Dysosomia**: distortion in the perception of a particular smell such as phantom olfactory stimulation.
- **Phantosmia**: perception of smells without olfactory stimulation.
- **Osmomotor disorders**: compulsive movements of lips, nostrils and tongue associated with epilepsy.
- **Olfactory 'Flashback'**: odours are recalled by the brain into the conscious mind.

Definitions of Relevant Terms

What is an Odour?

An odour is the volatile emission of a substance which can be perceived by the sense of smell. A scientific description of an odour is not actually possible, although one can use a collection of adjectives to communicate the experience of smelling a certain odour. An odour has a particular scent, with unique qualities, and whereas it is possible to categorize sounds, for example by notes or chords, it is not always possible to do the same with odours as each has its own distinct identity.

For most people, perception of an odour leads automatically to the conscious thought of it being either good or bad. The term odour, when used in perfumery, relates mostly to raw materials such as aromatic plants or essential oils. The term *odoriferous* usually refers to a substance giving out a pleasant odour.

How to Define Odours

Odours can be assessed by their strength or weakness, their tenacity or volatility, their lightness or intensity, their permanence or briefness.

Essential oils are fluids that come in various densities. Generally, the thinner the essential oil, the more volatile, for example Eucalyptus. However, the thicker, more viscous oils, such as Patchouli and Vetivert, tend to have more lingering smells. There is more than one odour in an individual essential oil – for example, although the dominant scent may be floral, it could also have an underlying spiciness. It is vital to learn how to develop olfactory discrimination in order to recognize the subtler odorant components found in a fragrance. Many factors such as humidity, room temperature, confinement or presence of other smells in the room can distort odours. For example, in a hot, tropical climate such as Singapore, a lesser quantity of essential oils will be required as the humidity tends to magnify and distort the overall smell.

Professional perfumers work in 'smell-free rooms' and do not consume strong, smelly foods, such as garlic or onions, which would distort their sense of smell. A common cold would also have a detrimental effect on their ability to smell. Certain extraction procedures, such as distillation, will also distort the original scent of a plant, mostly by intensifying it. Vaporizing essential oils in an unventilated room will saturate the air with odorant molecules and can make the air 'sickly'. It is therefore important to ventilate the room where the Aromatherapist works.

How to Refine the Sense of Smell

The first stage is to become aware of the many components in smells.

How we perceive or 'feel' certain smells is often determined by the following:

- The individual power of perception.
- Previous associations, including likes or dislikes.

- Whether the place where smelling takes place is already saturated by other smells; to enhance smelling, the room should be free of other odours.

The Traditional Approach to Blending

Simon Piesse, a perfumer-chemist, wrote a book entitled *The History of Perfume*, in which he explored the findings of his studies regarding the relationship between odour volatility and the sense of smell. He was interested in the physiological action of odours on the olfactive receptors and observed the differences generated by different types of smells.

A smell with a reasonably pleasant odour will stimulate the olfactory nerve endings and induce an emotional sensation. On the other hand, a smell with an aggressive odour will irritate the olfactory nerve endings and produce a reaction which is more akin to being physically hit. Furthermore, odours seem to affect the olfactive nerves at a particular pitch, just as sounds affect the ears. Certain odours, by the nature of their similarity, easily harmonize together. The harmony between Lemon, Lime, Orange and Verbena creates a higher octave of odours. There are also semi-odours (similar to half notes or half tones) such as Rose, Geranium and Neroli. At the other end of the scale there are scents such as Patchouli, Sandalwood and Vetivert, which easily harmonize together but have a low volatility, and as a result are perceived by the olfactory receptors at a lower octave.

Some of the natural perfumes of flowers greatly resemble those of others, so that they tend to be confused with each other. A common phenomenon with naturally occurring odours is that once they interact with the air, their scent changes to the extent that they are intensified or distorted. Piesse studied the degree and speed of evaporation or volatility of essential oils, combined with the resultant olfactory response. He related speed of evaporation to the distance a musical sound will travel and what effect it will have on the olfactory sense, for example, how quickly it will be perceived or how subtle or hard its effect. He then compared various smells to musical notes and chords. He divided the scent of essential oils into three main groups: **top** of the range, **middle** of the range and **base** or bottom of the range. It is now traditional to associate perfume components with this musical classification and to blend them in harmony with each other:

- *Top note*, or top of the range, is the *head note*. These are the most volatile scents and go straight to the head.
- *Middle note*, or middle of the range, is the *heart note* of a scent. This group of scents is not so volatile and after reaching the nose will soon travel down to the chest.
- *Base note*, or bottom of the range, is what gives a scent its *body note*. These scents evaporate very slowly and are often deeply penetrating and tenacious. Many scents from this group will chemically react with and 'fix' other scents. They are usually referred to as *fixatives of perfumes*.

Different groups or 'octaves' of scents have a tendency to react in a certain way with each other. The art of blending is to know how to choose and add scents and harmonize them together in 'odorant chords'. As the range of combinations is infinite it is easy to understand why making perfumes is both an art and a highly individual skill.

Aromatic Scents Terminology

Perfumers use specific terms to help them 'draw a sketch' of what sort of perfume they wish to create. Some of them relate to the type of odours to be used and some are descriptive adjectives of the effects these odours have on people. The following terms are used to describe the range of aromatic scents: floral, balsamic, fruity, smoky, wood, spicy, green (fern), herbal, musty, musky, pungent (almost repulsive).

There are five specific families of perfumes, which have been created:

1. Floral.
2. Leather (smoke, tobacco scent).
3. Fresh (green or mossy; can include citruses).
4. Ferns.
5. Amber or exotic smells.

The following words are often used to describe a perfume or its wearer: light, seductive, warm, moving, exotic, mysterious, vivaceous, tender, sharp, child-like, delicately unusual, romantic, provocative, powerful, radiant, voluptuous, distinguished, feminine, masculine, sophisticated, refined, enigmatic, sensuous, tenacious.

CHAPTER 6
The Applications of Aromatherapy

HISTORICAL DEVELOPMENT OF AROMATHERAPY

Henna the spikenard plants,
spikenard with saffron,
Calamus and cinnamon with all the chief
spices.
Thou are the fountain of the gardens,
A well of living waters,
And flowing streams from Lebanon.
The Song of Solomon

The methods of extracting herbal essences from aromatic plants were passed down to the Ancient Egyptians via the Assyrians and Babylonians, who themselves received this art from the very earliest civilizations of India, but the true origins are lost in the mists of time.

In China, the use of medicinal plants and acupuncture was recorded in 2800BC. Among the plants named as remedies were Aniseed, Cinnamon and Ginger. In India, *Ayurveda* (Brahma's sacred book on plants) names aromatic plants as part of the 'secret of eternal youth'. It also notes how it is possible to anaesthetize with the help of some plants, and gives advice for hygiene and health using aromatic plants.

The Sumerians (*c.*4000BC) used aromatic plants such as Fennel, Galbanum and Pine, a fact noted on clay tablets discovered in Syria in 1973. These tablets also contain the first written formulas for plant remedies.

In Ancient Egypt, around 3000BC, it was common practice to treat body, mind and soul with aromatic plants. The Egyptians were experts at making perfumes and cosmetics, and their knowledge was much in demand throughout the Mediterranean. Some of the aromatic plants used were: Aniseed, Cinnamon, Cardamom, Cumin, Frankincense, Bay, Mint and Myrrh. The legendary beauty of Queen Nefertiti was attributed to a skin lotion made from the oil of orchids and honey. Her baths were reputed to be scented with more than eighty different herbs and oils. The Egyptians also seemed to be well acquainted with the idea of 'as above, so below' and had already established the relationship between many plants and some of the heavenly bodies. They knew a lot about the influence that the Moon and the Sun had on life on Earth, and used this knowledge to balance the effects of the higher on the lower.

The word perfume comes from the Latin and literally means 'through the smoke', originally applying to fumigation. The perfumes of plants have been used for all sorts of reasons through the ages, but in particular to induce a state of mind that is open to contact with the spirit. For example, the priestesses of the Delphic Oracle would inhale 'holy fumes' (aromatic scents and sulphuric vapours) in order to reach a state of prophetic inspiration.

In many such rituals the smoke of aromatic herbs rising from small braziers was regarded as a means of communication between the visible world and the spiritual (invisible) world. Henbane, Mandragore, Sandalwood and sulphur vapours were commonly used as powerful narcotics which sent the seers into a state of trance which facilitated prophetic visions and healing. There was a hierarchy of smells, with pleasant smells being the attributes of holiness, while foul smells denoted the presence of evil. Diseases like the plague were believed to be carried by foul vapours, and so were given a burning reception of herbs and spices in the hope of dispersing them. The preparation of remedies was at first relatively crude, usually consisting of drying and crushing the leaves of plants, but as time went by it became more sophisticated.

In later Europe, the tradition of herbal medicine was kept alive in the monasteries and religious houses and the country folklore of different areas. In 1653, the great English herbalist, Nicholas Culpeper, published his classic encyclopaedia, listing the properties of many hundreds of plants, and the uses of their oils.

By the 17th and 18th Centuries, natural medicine had reached a high degree of sophistication. Antiseptics, tranquillizers, antipyretics, diuretics and analgesics were all in common use for several centuries before modern science discovered how they worked. There is strong evidence to suggest that throughout history people have tried to unravel the mystery of smell, exploring the great range of essential oils available to them. Through trial and error, it has been recorded that these scents can ease pain, awaken feelings, heal the body, calm fears and stimulate the mind. Using Aromatherapy leads to a voyage of discovery – or, rather, one of 'self-discovery'.

METHODS OF APPLICATION OF ESSENTIAL OILS

The popular perception of Aromatherapy is that it consists of a nice gentle massage with a pleasantly scented oil, and that it will promote an hour or so of relaxation and peace, with the promise that the nice smells will work magic on the body's systems and health will return almost immediately. In some cases this is true, it does seem to work this way, but Aromatherapy has far more to offer. I was fortunate to be born in the Alps and I grew up with the notion that if you were unwell but not acutely ill, before you went to the doctor you would try an appropriate herbal tisane or remedy, usually obtained from the local pharmacy. You had to be fairly ill to make the visit to the doctor, and, once there, the doctor would often recommend the same remedies after having established that the problem did not require more drastic measures. So, interestingly, the revival of complementary and holistic medicine is really about 'going back' fifty years or so. It encourages a more gentle form of treatment for health problems, using natural remedies before unleashing powerful chemicals into the body. My uncle, a homeopathic doctor from whom I learned a great deal, always said of pharmaceutical remedies that they are like 'using a gun to kill a fly', sometimes resulting in further damage to the rest of the organism.

Caution Regarding the Use of Essential Oils

Essential oils are safe so long as safety guidance, application procedures and dosage are respected. Some essential oils are easier and safer to use than others. It is important to follow instructions when self-prescribing in order to obtain the best results and avoid unnecessary discomfort.

If preparing a treatment for children, pregnant women or people with medical conditions, the first thing to do is decide whether Aromatherapy is suitable for this situation. After choosing safe essential oils with the right therapeutic benefits, it is always better to start with a weaker blend and add more essential oil at the next treatment if necessary.

Which Application Method is Best?

Massage is undoubtedly the most efficient way in which to help the body recover from stress and illness, as well as regenerating the whole being. However, sometimes it is not appropriate or possible to use massage and a different approach is necessary. Also, it is not always easy to perform self-massage or to have someone handy who can do so, and therefore other methods of application may be more suitable to treat problems on a day-to-day basis.

Only the most important methods are listed below, along with the most useful carriers in which essential oils can be diluted, for safe and easy application.

1. Air Diffusion, Vaporization and Inhalation

Inhalation occurs naturally when we breathe, but we can consciously chose to inhale essential oils to bring about therapeutic changes in our body. Usually, it is best either to use a tissue or to put a drop on a pillow at night, as the essential oils are very strong when they are undiluted.

Steam Inhalation

This method does not require any apparatus, just a bowl of steaming hot water and the essential oils.

Adults Please note that this is not necessarily a good method for asthma sufferers as it can aggravate the condition. Add five to six drops of essential oils to 4 pints of water, stand over the steam (as close as is comfortable) and cover your head and the bowl with a towel. Breathe in steam through your mouth and nose. This is excellent for chest and nasal congestion, for the treatment of oily facial skin and to absorb essential oils into the system.

Children This method is not suitable for children under five in case they should suddenly knock over the bowl of steaming water. Children should not be left unattended near the hot water. Add two drops of essential oils only and ensure that the child is not standing too close to the water as they may find the steam overwhelming. Remove the bowl away from children when the treatment is complete.

Essential Oils Diffusers

There are three main types of device which allow diffusion of essential oils into the air, and in principle all have a beneficial effect upon the air and can prevent the spread of airborne diseases like the flu. However, it must be pointed out that none of them were designed to be used for long periods. Having used all of them myself, I can also see some of the drawbacks.

Electrical Diffuser This is a device which appeared a good few years ago. It has an elaborate small glass receptacle which is connected to a little motor. Its purpose is to diffuse the oils and to purify the air. These electrical devices are the most powerful and should be used only a few times a day, for very short periods (15 minutes is probably enough).

Traditional Candle Burner The power of the candle underneath the small water bowl is a lot fiercer than is often assumed. Although an efficient means of keeping odours and smoke at bay in a social situation, it should only be used for short periods of time. The reason is that after a short while some of the less volatile chemicals from the essential oils (like gums and resins) will begin to 'cook up' the oils and give off subtle, unpleasant fumes which will saturate the air. These have been found to give many people a severe headache. I have also found these burners to be dangerous around children and pets and I know of some nasty accidents, so they must be placed somewhere where they cannot do any damage.

Portable Humidifier This device is fairly safe and very effective, especially for asthma sufferers where a special compartment is included to put the oils in. But, again, as the oils evaporate with the heat and water, a thick oily residue forms, getting into the container and clogging it. After about a month or so of regular use this device is likely to become less efficient.

Choice and Dosage of Essential Oils

Recommendation: only one or two oils should be used at a time; *only one to three drops of essential oils are needed each time.* It is best to choose essential oils which are light and evaporate easily, such as citruses or peppermint, to avoid making the air too heavy. Always clean the device between uses. If using any of the devices to prevent the spread of infectious diseases then the time they are in use should be controlled.

What are the Benefits to be Obtained from Inhalation and Vaporization?

• Keeps the air clean and fresh. It is particularly good when working in offices, air-conditioned places and around people who smoke. With smokers, this method should be used in conjunction with an air ionizer.

• Good for keeping diseases at bay, such as infantile disorders, flu viruses, Legionnaire's Disease, and possibly even meningitis and TB.

• Helps with stress by relaxing the mind and creating a happier mood, thus preventing a lot of stress-related problems; creates a generally healthier environment in which to live.

2. Body Massage

If you are fortunate to have someone to hand who can give you a massage with essential oils, in the comfort of your own home then you are very lucky. However, you can give yourself head, face, hands, feet and leg massage without problems. The percentage of essential oils to carrier remains the same.

Different Styles of Massage for Different Needs

What are the benefits of a light, fast massage and a slow, deep massage? A light and fast massage, such as Swedish massage, activates the processes regulated by the sympathetic nervous system. Swedish massage is not considered a very healing and relaxing technique by many Aromatherapists. It is best used in the context of sports massage and before exercise at the gym. It releases stamina and energy and encourages bodily excretion.

A slow, deep massage, such as lymphatic massage, will activate the processes regulated by the parasympathetic nervous system and will tend to induce a state of mild hypnosis. More holistic than Swedish massage, it permits both the mind and body to relax and therefore promotes healing at a much deeper level. It will help psychosomatic conditions through deep release of stress and helps sleep patterns.

Mixing Instructions for a Full Body Massage for Adults

A full body massage will require about 30ml of carrier oil. The average amount of essential oils to be added will be three to four drops per 10ml; for 30ml, three × four = twelve drops altogether.

Sesame Oil Specially recommended for sport massage, stiff joints, rheumatism and fluid retention.

For a Local Massage Six to seven drops per 10ml (particularly when treating muscle and joint problems).

For a Facial Massage One to two drops per 10ml of carrier oil; recommended carrier oil is apricot or peach kernel with the addition of jojoba or avocado.

For Child's Massage Under the age of five – three drops per 20ml. From five to twelve years five drops in 20ml of carrier oil. Choose oils suitable for children. Sweet almond oil is the best carrier, and you can add 20 per cent of olive oil if the skin is very dry. You can also add wheatgerm or avocado oil in the blend.

For Pregnancy Two drops per 10ml of carrier oil, making sure that you include about ten drops of wheatgerm oil and ten drops of avocado. Any carrier can be used.

3. Aromatic Bath

It is common practice to put drops of essential oils into the bath. While this is the quickest way to reap the benefits of inhalation, it does not in my mind constitute a proper aromatic bath.

Certainly, no more than four or five drops of the chosen essential oil should be used, and this method does not apply to children because it could cause skin and eye irritation.

The Art of the Aromatic Bath

The aromatic bath is very old; in Ancient Egypt women used to take an aromatic bath two to three times daily, followed by a steam bath, believing this would prolong youth and longevity. Aromatic baths are the most efficient way to administer a very potent home treatment, as they give instant benefits, or they can provide the perfect follow-up from a visit to the Aromatherapist.

Another advantage is that the combined effect of the warm water with the blended essential oils will regenerate the surface layers of the skin and provide relief for skin ailments. Meanwhile, inhalation of the scent from the essential oils will work on the central nervous system and cause a dynamic reaction, often resulting in interesting healing breakthroughs.

The procedures for blending are the same as preparing a massage blend. The essential oils should be selected by looking them up in the therapeutic property table or consulting the table of ailments.

It is important to note that the treatment should be made fresh everyday, unless a formula has been specifically prepared for you by your Aromatherapist.

For a Full Body Application About 30ml of carrier oil are needed for an application to the whole body (if you are smaller than average, use a little bit less). Choose from a maximum of four different essential oils. The more oils you use, the more saturated the blend will become; while the end result may be most pleasant, it could equally be rather discordant, so err on the side of caution.

55

Number of Drops As already mentioned, only three to four drops should be added for every 10ml of carrier oil, giving a total of ten to twelve drops altogether. A stronger dosage may be required when making a local application for problems such as muscular aches, arthritis or painful cramps. It should reach no more than twenty drops and should not be applied near the face.

A hot, short bath (about 10 minutes) is more suitable in the day as it gives energy, while a warm, longer bath (around 20 minutes) is better at night because it is more sedative. Of course, the choice of essential oils will reinforce those tendencies.

4. Face Mask Made with Fine Clay

Clay is a natural product with many benefits for the skin. It has special medicinal properties due to its structure and large mineral-salt content. Its amazing healing properties can help many difficult skin disorders such as psoriasis or acute eczema. It is antiseptic, purifying, re-mineralizing, mildly exfoliating and can help regulate the secretions of sebaceous glands and so is recommended for dandruff, oily skin and acne (and also for dry skin conditions). French white clay and green clay are very good to use, not only for face masks but for all types of skin care.

How to Use

Mix the clay with a little bit of warm water to make it into a paste and add the essential oils, which have been previously diluted in a carrier oil such avocado oil, sweet almond oil or apricot kernel oil. Make sure you stir the paste thoroughly. Apply to the face or any area of the body which suffers from psoriasis or dermatitis. Leave it on for 15 to 20 minutes while relaxing. Remove it with warm water and repeat the treatment weekly.

5. Creams and Ointments

Aqueous Base Cream or Lotion

A vegetable emulsion, preferably free of animal products or pesticides, makes a good neutral base cream to which essential oils can be added and used easily. This method is more appropriate for facial skin conditions that are caused by excess sebum secretion, and it is also easier to use when dealing with children's skin ailments.

The lotion is made of the same ingredient as the cream, but it is made deliberately thinner than a cream. It is more suitable for massaging the hands and feet as it quickly disappears, leaving the skin smooth and not too greasy. Avocado oil, aloe vera gel, jojoba, rosehip oil and wheatgerm can all be added to the cream or lotion to enrich them. Only a small quantity of essential oils is required in a face cream as they are so concentrated. Overuse of essential oils can cause skin damage.

Arnica Ointment (Latin name: Arnica montana*)*

Arnica is a hairy herbaceous plant which grows in mountainous areas above 800 metres. The word 'arnica' is said to be derived from the word *ptarmica* (to sneeze) and the powder of its flowers does make you sneeze. Hildegard de Bingen refers to it as the 'herb for falls' and recommends that it be used in compresses and decoctions. In the 18th Century, arnica seemed to have been a popular tincture, and was recommended for 'bumps and knocks'.

Therapeutic Properties Arnica is renowned for its anti-bruising properties, but it is equally efficient with swelling, sprains and concussion. It is anti-inflammatory and has strong healing properties. It is also renowned for its restorative and decongestant effect on the venous system and is traditionally used for broken capillary vessels.

Uses It is found as the main ingredient in: creams used in sports for bruises or sprains; massage creams for severe fluid retention particularly in the legs; and for mature and blotchy skin care cream.

Calendula Ointment or Cream (Latin name: Calendula officinalis)

The ointment, the cream or fixed oil are obtained by macerating the bright orange flower heads of the French marigold. The cream is a water-based emulsion which is nongreasy and is more suitable for 'acne-like conditions'. The ointment is made mostly from beeswax and can be used for healing, or as a protective film where the skin may be damaged. The ointment is very useful for treating grazes or ulcers.

Therapeutic Properties The cream or ointment is cicatrisant, anti-inflammatory, promotes fast skin cell growth, is vulnerary, emollient and anti-pruritic.

Hypericum Ointment (Latin name: Hypericum perforatum)

This ointment is made in a similar manner to the Calendula ointment. It is also anti-inflammatory, anti-pruritic, cicatrisant and anti-neuralgic.

6. Compresses

Compresses require a bowl of boiling water, sterile gauze or lint from the chemist and, of course, essential oils. Add five to six drops of the desired essential oils to 4 pints of boiling water. Skim the surface with a sterile gauze –

hot or cold compresses can be used, depending upon the ailment:

- Hot compresses can be applied to abscesses, cuts, grazes, acne, boils, skin infections, chest infections with mucus and rheumatism.
- Cold compresses still require boiling the water and adding the oils while the water is hot, then letting it cool down. Cold compresses are needed with fever, sprains, muscular tears, spasms, bruises, arthritis, joint inflammation and swelling, nerve inflammation, oedema and varicose veins.

7. Hip or Foot Bath

This requires about 4 pints of boiling water with seven to eight drops of essential oils added. Immerse the parts to be treated. It is suitable for thrush, cystitis, poor circulation, chilblains, athlete's foot (with 50 per cent malt vinegar added to the water). The treatment for athlete's foot will be more complete if a cream or ointment containing essential oils is used afterwards.

8. Sitz Bath

This is useful for cystitis after labour. It requires warm water and three drops of essential oils to a pint of water. If stitches are present, using an ointment afterwards will help recovery.

CARRIER OILS

Carrier oils are vegetable oils, otherwise described as 'fixed' oils. They should be 100 per cent pure, unrefined vegetable oils. With the genetically modified foods alert, carrier oils must be of organic sources and processed by the 'cold pressed' method. Carrier oils are excellent for lubricating the skin, facilitating a smooth, flowing massage, and are also used to dissolve the essential oils and thus control the strength of the treatment. There are many different vegetable oils which can be used as carrier oils, or that can be added to the main carrier to increase its moisturizing and regenerative power.

Viscosity is a term which relates to the density or thickness of a vegetable oil. Different carrier oils have different densities; they can be light and fluid with an almost water-like quality, or thick enough to provide a protective film for the skin.

With massage, the thicker the oil the deeper the massage; conversely the lighter the oil the more superficial. The choice of essential oils will also contribute to the end result.

Main Carrier Oils and Gels for Massage

Note: Nut oils should not be used on nut allergy sufferers

(Sweet) Almond Oil (Latin name: Prunus amygdalus var. dulcis)

The name *Amygdalus* means almond. The tree originates from central Asia, and is cultivated in Mediterranean countries and California. The oil is extracted from the seed of the almond tree, which is generally classified as an almond nut.

Therapeutic Properties This oil contains many vitamins: vitamin A (retinol), vitamins B1, B2, B3, B5 and B6. It has anti-stretch mark, anti-wrinkle, anti-aging, regenerative and emollient properties and is widely used in dermatology and cosmetic products. It keeps the skin supple and elastic. Sweet almond oil is used particularly for baby skin care. It is also recommended for dry skin and can be added to: nourishing night creams; lip balms; moisturizing hand creams; eye contour creams and mature skin creams.

Aloe Vera Gel

There are about 180 types of aloes, but the official pharmaceutical aloe is *Aloe ferox*. In Indonesia, aloes are named 'crocodile tongue' because of their prickly teeth around the edges of the leaves. The gel is extracted from the plant *Aloe vera*. It is mainly collected in the Cape in South Africa and Kenya. It grows 2 to 3 metres high and originally came from arid deserts, surviving in dry and scorching heats. Interestingly, it is the most effective natural medicine for skin burns. *Aloe vera* itself is a cultivated plant, a cousin of *Aloe ferox*, and, being cultivated, is the only aloe which is not on the endangered species list.

Known Therapeutic Uses This plant has been used as an anti-inflammatory, an aperitif, an emmenagogue, a laxative, a prophylactic and more recently has been found to be extraordinarily healing for skin burns or any problematic skin diseases.

Therapeutic Properties Aloe vera is soothing, cooling, moisturizing, regenerative and rehydrating and seems to suit all skin conditions. Because of this, it is often added to cosmetic formulations.

Application It can be used on its own or blended with other base creams as it mixes easily and gives the other creams or ointments a silky, smooth quality. The following ailments particularly benefit from aloe vera gel in an aromatic cream formula: heat rash, nappy rash, shaving rash, eczema, severe skin inflammation, skin infections, grazes, sunburn (with Lavender or Tea Tree) and ordinary burns.

Grapeseed Oil

Grapeseed oil comes from the Red Vine, Latin name *Vitis vinifera*, bot.: *Vitaceae*.

The Red Vine has been cultivated since ancient times around the Mediterranean basin for its wine. Grape seeds contain a variable quantity of lipids (5 to 20 per cent). The oil is used in dietetics for frying and seasoning as it is a light oil, rich in linoleic acid. The following fatty acids are contained in grapeseed oil: linoleic, oleic, palmitic and stearic.

Linoleic acid is an essential fatty acid that is important for the health of the skin and the cell membranes. Grapeseed oil is known to be regenerative, moisturizing and emollient. It has very little smell, and, as it is not a nut, can be used on people who are allergic to nuts.

Apricot Kernel (Latin name: Prunus armenica)

Apricot is a rather small fruit tree which grows wild from Iran right across to Manchuria. It was introduced by the Romans and Arabs into the countries they conquered. It was mentioned in Arabian medicine as a cure for haemorrhoids, aching noses and earache. Its fruit was said to symbolize the female sexual organs and countless love potions and philtres claimed that adding the pulp or oil from the apricot would arouse passion. Nowadays, it is commonly used as a regenerative, nourishing and softening beauty mask. Its sweet kernel produces a very fine oil that is particularly good for facial massage.

Therapeutic Properties Apricot kernel oil is a very light oil which has emollient, purifying, nourishing and regenerative skin properties. It is often used in bath oils, and face and body massage oils for all skin types.

Hazelnut Oil (Latin name: Corys avellana)

Its name is derived from the Greek *corys*, meaning helmet, because the shape of its shell resembles that of the helmets of Ancient Greek soldiers. The hazel tree grows in Europe, western and central Asia and north Africa, and is very common in woods, copses, hedges and low mountains. The hazelnut is an ovoid fruit which contains two seeds at the beginning of its growth but usually only one of them will develop fully into a hazelnut.

Hazel sticks are still used by dowsers or water diviners to find underground water springs. Sorcerers used to call for rain by thrashing ponds with hazel sticks and magic wands are traditionally made of hazel wood.

Therapeutic Properties Hazelnut oil has softening, moisturizing and regenerative properties. It helps prevent dehydration and has anti-aging properties. It is not as regenerative as Sweet Almond, but nevertheless can be used as a replacement for it. Hazelnut particularly improves the corneum layer on the surface of the skin.

Olive Oil (Latin name: Olea europaea)

The olive tree grows in the Mediterranean area but is also common in Asia and Africa. The olive tree is valued for its leaves, fruit and oil. Properly prepared, olives are rich in minerals and vitamins. People traditionally used the first cold-pressed oil as a softening agent to prevent sunburn. It also has laxative and vermifuge properties. The leaf has febrifuge properties and is used in Corsica and the south of France to lower blood pressure and cholesterol.

The olive tree was revered in Greek mythology and the most sacred olive tree grew in Minerva's temple. The olive tree is a symbol of peace, and in the Bible Noah is offered an

59

olive branch by the dove. The expression 'offering an olive branch' refers to offering peace.

Therapeutic Properties The leaf of the olive tree is known to be hypotensive, vasodilatory, hypoglycaemic, anti-cholesterol and regulates heartbeat. It also is antispasmodic, sedative, digestive and has diuretic and anti-diabetic properties. The oil is anti-inflammatory, cooling and healing. It is also good for eczema, inflamed skin, arthritis, gout and dry scalp problems. It can be included in eye contour creams and regenerative treatments for stressed and damaged skin.

Peach Kernel Oil (Latin name: Prunus persica*)*

Persicus means Persia, the country thought to be the birthplace of the peach tree. Known in China in 20BC, the peach tree is commonly cultivated all over the warmer part of Europe and the Mediterranean basin. Hundreds of varieties exist, ranging from the 'furry' skinned peach to smooth-skinned nectarines.

Therapeutic Properties The oil tones and soothes the skin, and is a gentle exfoliator and moisturizer. Is very good for facial and neck massage and creams.

Sesame (Latin name: Sesamum indicum, *Bot. Pedaliaceae)*

Sesame has many names: in Sanskrit it is *Tila,* in Malay *Widjin,* in Chinese *Moa* and in Japanese *Koba*. Sesame is an herbaceous plant from tropical and subtropical countries. It is widely cultivated in China, India, Turkey and the Gulf. Sesame oil is extracted from the seeds of the herbaceous plant. The plant contains many seeds that are oval and flattened; the most common ones are white.

Sesame is purported to contain legendary power to reveal hidden treasures, secret ways or to open locked doors.

Sesame is used a lot in Indian medicine for disorders of the joints, for lymphatic problems and as an expectorant for chest congestion. It is a very viscose but healing massage oil. It warms the body, decreases swelling of the muscles, and gives a rhythmic, flowing massage. It is good for aging skin, the hair and scalp, but is not often used in Aromatherapy because it is fairly 'oily'. It has a strong nutty smell.

Therapeutic Properties This oil is remarkably stable as it contains the natural anti-oxidizing agents sesamol and sesaminol. It also contains many fatty acids: linoleic, oleic, palmitic and stearic. Fatty acids merge easily with the strata corneum and regenerate the top layer of the skin.

Like many of the carrier oils it is used in dermatology and in cosmetic products. It has emollient and moisturizing properties similar to olive oil, but it does not oxidize so easily. It is also very helpful when giving a deep massage as it is more viscose than other oils. It can be used to treat fluid retention, swollen joints, arthritis, rheumatism and oedema.

Vegetable Oils that Can be Added to the Main Carrier

Avocado (Latin name: Laurus persea*)*

Originating from tropical America, the Avocado tree can reach 5 to 15 metres high. This tree is very commonly cultivated. Several varieties are marketed, notably from Mexico and Israel. In America, the Avocado tree is mostly cultivated in California and Florida.

The word avocado is a Spanish rendering of the Aztec *ahua guati*; the Aztecs also referred to it as the 'tree with testicles' as they believed it to be an aphrodisiac food. They used it both as food and to make their hair grow.

Avocado oil is extracted from the fruit of the Avocado tree. The fruit and the oil contain fructose and glucose (currently used in many skincare products) and lipids and it is rich in vitamins, especially vitamins A and D.

Therapeutic Properties Avocado oil is an ingredient found in many healing creams because of its vitamin D and potassium content. It is said to have soothing, astringent, moisturizing and regenerative properties and to be efficient for eczema and very dry skin. It offers protection to the face in poor weather conditions.

The oil can be used in aromatic preparations for the face, body, hands and feet, care and for loss of hair, alopecia or to treat damaged hair.

It can also be added to cold creams to make up night creams for damaged, mature, dry or sensitive skin. It is entirely safe to use on children and babies. It is often added to a lighter carrier oil.

Jojoba (Latin name: Simmondsia chinensis*)*

The word jojoba derives from its Ancient Mexican name *chochoba*. It grows in semi-desert areas in northern Mexico, Arizona and California. It is now widely cultivated in South America, Israel and Africa. The Mexican Indians made a drink with Jojoba to induce states of hallucination and visions.

Jojoba seed can yield up to 60 per cent oil. Californian Indians used it to fight cancer and Mexican Indians used it to fortify the hair, but its essential virtue was to preserve a soft skin.

Therapeutic Properties Jojoba is used in dermatological preparations for eczema, acne, psoriasis, dermatitis and dandruff. Jojoba oil has notable emollient, regenerative, astringent and tonic properties. It stimulates hair growth and has natural hair-conditioning properties. It can be used in an Aromatherapy hair blend by itself of with 50 per cent olive oil.

Rose Hip (Latin name: Rosa rubiginosa*)*

This is a rose bush which grows up to 2 metres high. The flowers produce a bright red oval fruit which remains on the bush throughout the winter. Rose is believed to have magic love powers and was used by sorcerers to make love potions. It is also used for divination and is renowned for its healing properties.

Therapeutic Properties It is rich in lipids (about 8 per cent) and fatty acids. Rose Hip is efficient to treat burns and bad scarring.

Rose Hip oil is known to promote healthy regrowth of skin cell and to delay skin aging. It is softening, moistening and forms a protective film over the skin. While mostly used for facial massage and creams, it can also be used for any scar tissue on the body.

Wheatgerm (Latin name: Triticum vulgare*)*

Wheatgerm oil is obtained from the fresh wheat germ. It is very rich in vitamin E, but is expensive and does not keep for very long. It has a strong smell and goes rancid easily.

Therapeutic Properties Often added to other oils for its healing properties, Wheatgerm is recommended to prevent stretch marks and for dehydrated and devitalized skins. Can be used in pregnancy for abdominal massage and also blended with other carriers.

Witch Hazel (Latin name: Hamamelis virginiana*)*

Very common in North America, Witch Hazel grows in the damp forests from Mississippi all the way to Canada. This tree resembles a hazel tree.

Its name is related to the fact that it projects its seeds rather violently and as a result people believed that the plant was bewitched.

Therapeutic Properties The distilled water or gel are astringent, analgesic and vasoconstricting, making it an excellent medicine for veins. It has homeostatic, anti-inflammatory, anti-pruritic and antibacterial properties.

The distilled water can be used as a carrier for essential oils when dealing with cuts, stings, wounds, shaving rash, burns and infected or inflamed skin.

In a 100ml solution, add 50 per cent Witch Hazel distilled water, 50 per cent Rose distilled water and a maximum of twenty drops of essential oils to make either an aftershave lotion or a deodorant.

SAFETY GUIDELINES ON THE USE OF ESSENTIAL OILS

Once you have bought your oils from a reliable specialist supplier, there are a few points you should observe to safeguard the quality and therapeutic power of your essential oils. As the rule, the correct way to store your essential oils is to keep them away from the air, light or heat.

You should ensure that they are stored in appropriate containers, such as dark glass bottles, are well capped or sealed, and are away from light or heat to avoid evaporation, oxidation and damaging activity from sunlight. They should also have a dropper insert in the inside of the cap for easy use when pouring out drops. You should avoid leaving them by a window or a heater, where again sunlight or heat can affect them. Once your essential oils are blended with vegetable, the blend will go rancid very quickly, about a month afterwards.

Lifespan of Essential Oils

Essential oils have a variable lifespan and usually the more volatile oils such as Lemon or Orange will deteriorate much quicker than less volatile oils such as Vetivert. In general, all citruses are very volatile and do not like heat as it makes them decay faster. The rate of evaporation of the herb group of essential oils is variable, as some are highly volatile while others are far less so, as is easily demonstrated by the differences in lifespan between Lavender and Sandalwood: Lavender will last about six months, Sandalwood about eighteen months if stored properly. Essential oils from gums, woods or roots are known to have very low volatility and do not evaporate so easily, and as a result have a longer lifespan as can be seen with Sandalwood, Cedarwood and Myrrh.

To Use Your Oils Safely and Efficiently You Need to Read the Following:

Essential oils are very concentrated and, like most chemical substances, they are potentially dangerous if misused. When using your essential oils the same rules of safety apply as when using any pharmaceutical remedy.

First you should always read the name on the label before pouring the oil out. Secondly, if you are not sure what an oil can be used for, either find out from a reliable source or abstain altogether. The list on page 72 is designed to highlight any safety issues and is there to help you choose your oils with care. Always remember to replace the cap immediately after use and put the oils back in a safe place. You should always keep the oils away from children and pets as the oils could cause harm if they were accidentally spilled and came into contact with the skin or eyes or found their way inside the body. Oil burners are a particular worry. Apart from possible burns from spillage, the essential oils tend to have non-volatile components such as gums and others, which remain after the initial evaporation of the lighter chemicals. The water in the small ball becomes overheated and the residue chemicals begin to give off fumes which can cause headaches.

Proper Care Must Be Taken before Using Essential Oils on Yourself or Others

If you wish to use essential oils for members of your family, you should take into account that different people have different degrees of sensitivity to chemicals and smells. Unless you are a properly qualified Aromatherapist, you should not attempt to diagnose or prescribe oils for others. The same applies to yourself; if you are feeling unusually unwell and don't know what's wrong, you should not attempt self-diagnosis but should see your doctor.

There are some factors that can affect a person's response to a treatment, such as being tired, upset, stressed, worried, and so on. Everyone is different and particular attention should be paid to the strength of each individual essential oil, as some of them are much stronger than others. Another relevant factor to take into account when assessing the strength of essential oils is the season or climate of the country in which you live. In the summer, or in a hot and humid climate, scents tend to expand and intensify and therefore affect people more strongly and their body will respond differently than in a cold climate. It is important to adjust the dosage to reflect these considerations.

Some essential oils should definitely not be used on young children, while others are better avoided until further research has been done. Some essential oils could also be very hazardous to pregnant women. Some oils can increase high blood pressure while others can decrease it, so if given to the wrong person could cause much trouble.

One more word of caution, taking essential oils internally (orally) should be avoided as this can result in the following: nausea, vertigo, convulsions, epilepsy, coma or even death.

If you were exposed through accidental spillage to aromatic vapours or have to work all day in a clinic where there is no direct ventilation the following could arise: headaches, nausea, disorientation, euphoria and later depletion of nervous energy. You should not practise Aromatherapy in confined spaces, especially if they do not have a window that you can open for ventilation. The air can become saturated with the smells and can make the therapist feel sick and tired.

Listed further down are some of the tendencies essential oils have and some of the hazards they can create. Some essential oils can be euphoric and can make you feel dizzy and disorientated; some are skin irritants and if used wrongly can damage your skin; some have strong emmenagogic properties and can bring on periods, which could interfere with pregnancy; some can bring on uterine contractions and are classified as abortifacient, which could lead to miscarriage.

Another caution, after inhaling or being treated with essential oils, it is always recommended that you drive with particular diligence, as the oils may have relaxed your reflexes more than you are accustomed to.

Skin irritation or dermal sensitization can also occur with some of the essential oils, so please consult the list about the hazards of individual essential oils. These problems are due to some of the chemical constituents contained within the oils.

Photosensitivity

Finally, essential oils (even when diluted), if applied to the skin can react adversely if exposed to direct sunlight or the ultraviolet light of sunbeds, causing permanent local pigmentation change or even skin cancer. In today's age of ozone layer depletion and major skin cancer alerts, it is a problem that must be taken very seriously. Some oils, Bergamot, for example, will allow very fast penetration of ultraviolet light, which will burn the underlayer of the skin, causing brown marks or worse. Note also that many of the citruses are very photosensitive.

The following is an alphabetical guide to using essential oils safely. Note that the listing only applies to external application and inhalation of essential oils.

Angelica It can increase photosensitivity and if used repeatedly and in quantity, it can be abortive. If adding to a blend, use more sparingly than other oils so that its own pungent smell does not overcome the blend. It is a strong oil.

Aniseed This is very powerful oil. It should be used in smaller quantities than other oils and only when it is absolutely needed. It is highly euphoric, can be toxic to the nervous system and should not be used on epileptics, in preg-

nancy, or on children and babies. It should not be used on anyone suffering from mastitis or breast cancer.

If adding to a blend, use more sparingly than other oils so that its own pungent smell does not overcome the blend.

Basil It is a powerful oil, which is also very euphoric. I have found it to cause headaches and nausea followed by emotional outbursts, nervous depletion and a sense of disorientation, even when used in small quantities. It does not agree with everyone, so caution is recommended.

If adding to a blend, use more sparingly than other oils so that its own pungent smell does not overcome the blend.

Benzoin Can increase photosensitivity.

Bergamot A major photosensitive oil; otherwise very safe to use.

Black Pepper This is a skin and mucous membrane irritant (especially the eyes), and should not be used on people with skin ailments, varicose veins, haemorrhoids or kidney disease.

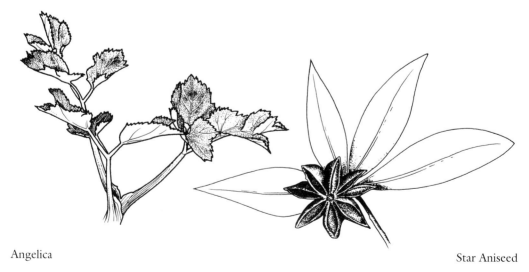

Angelica

Star Aniseed

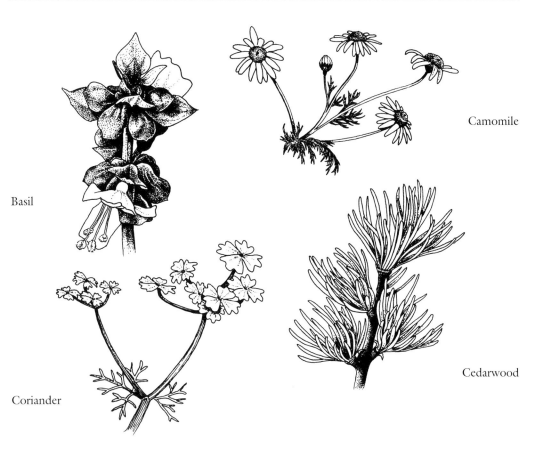

Basil

Camomile

Coriander

Cedarwood

Camomile Safe.

Cedarwood Should not be used on babies, children and pregnant women. It is toxic to the nervous system and can cause abortion.

Cinnamon Only the *leaf* should be used. It is a minor skin irritant. It is also an emmenagogue and can bring on uterine contractions, so is therefore potentially an abortifacient. Its use should be avoided where there is high blood pressure as it increases body heat and causes discomfort. It is a strong oil, which acts very quickly. If adding to a blend, use more sparingly than other oils so that its own pungent smell does not overcome the blend.

Clary Sage Inhaling can cause light-headedness, disorientation and slows down reflexes. It is a powerful nervine and myo-relaxant. It is an emmenagogue and should not be used on women suffering from mastitis or cancer of the reproductive system. Another powerful oil which can cause fast reactions.

If adding to a blend, use more sparingly than other oils so that its own pungent smell does not overcome the blend.

Coriander Used in therapeutic doses, it is safe.

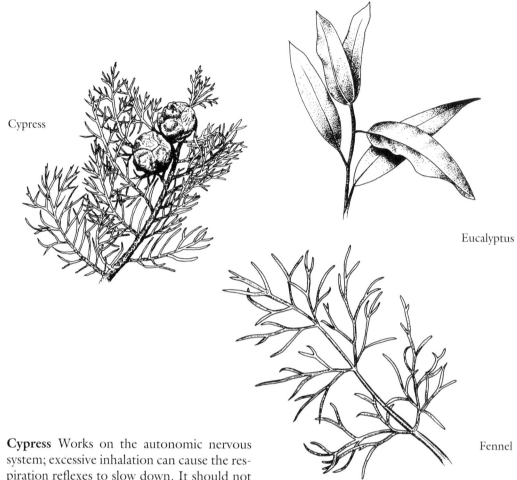

Cypress

Eucalyptus

Fennel

Cypress Works on the autonomic nervous system; excessive inhalation can cause the respiration reflexes to slow down. It should not be used on children under the age of five and women suffering from mastitis.

Eucalyptus Excessive prolonged use is not safe. It can cause nausea, vomiting and diarrhoea; it can also slow the respiratory reflexes. Taken internally, it can stop the breathing process. This oil should not be used on babies and children under five. It can damage the kidneys and so should not be used on anyone who suffers from kidney disease.

Fennel This should never be used on epileptics or people suffering from convulsions. It is not suitable for children under ten. Excessive inhalation can cause nausea and migraines and prolonged use can cause trembling. It should not be used in pregnancy and can cause abortions. A powerful oil with a quick action.

If adding to a blend, use more sparingly than other oils so that its own pungent smell does not overcome the blend.

Frankincense Excessive inhalation can cause light-headedness and mild disorientation, but it is fine in therapeutic doses. It is a very powerful oil which can unsettle people suffering from phobias or psychotic delusions.

Geranium Safe in therapeutic doses. If adding to a blend, use more sparingly than other oils so that its own pungent smell does not overcome the blend.

Ginger Used neat, it can irritate the skin and mucous membrane, particularly if used on people suffering from dermatitis, allergies or eczema. It can raise high blood pressure and increase body heat.

Grapefruit Can increase photosensitivity, but otherwise it is very safe.

Hyssop It only takes 2ml of Hyssop taken internally to cause epilepsy or even death, as this oil is a nervine poison. Inhaling too much can cause light-headedness, nausea and headaches. It is an emmenagogue and abortifacient. It should not be used on babies, children, pregnant women, the elderly and epileptics. It is a powerful oil, which I find difficult to use.

Jasmine As it is an absolute(petroleum solvent extraction, *see* methods of extraction), only the effect of its scent is considered. In therapeutic doses it is safe and its smell is very beneficial.

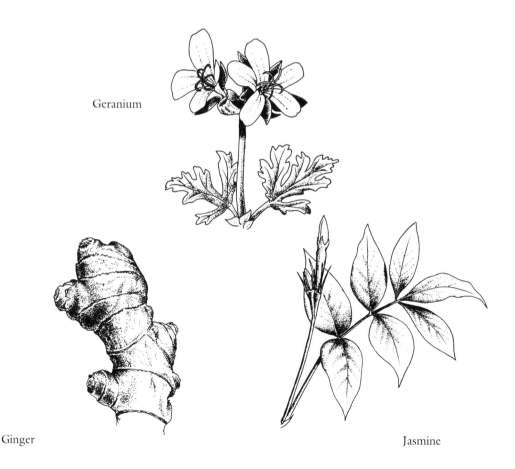

Geranium

Ginger

Jasmine

Juniper A fast-acting oil which should not be used when there is a kidney infection or kidney problems. It can cause kidney lesions, nephritis, stupor and sleepiness and can be dangerous in pregnancy. It is not suitable for babies and children. It should not be used for more than four to five weeks consecutively.

Lavender Can cause drowsiness in people sensitive to it. It can also trigger asthma fits on some people because of the strength of the pure essential oil. Otherwise, it is safe to use and can be used on babies, children, pregnant women, the elderly and the mentally handicapped.

Lemon It is an oil which, like Bergamot, can increase photosensitivity and can also be a skin irritant for people with a sensitive skin. It is a bit too strong to use on children under ten as it stings, but is safe to use in pregnancy.

Lemon Grass This can cause skin and mucous membrane irritation when applied neat or blended. If adding to a blend, use more sparingly than other oils so that its own pungent smell does not overcome the blend. A very powerful oil that should not be used on children under ten.

Lime Another photosensitive oil, but otherwise safe.

Marjoram This is a strong sedative that can cause drowsiness. It is a powerful hypotensive and diuretic and can cause kidney problems. If adding to a blend, use more sparingly than other oils so that its own pungent smell does not overcome the blend.

Melissa Safe to use on everyone in therapeutic doses.

Myrrh Safe to use in pregnancy and with children over two.

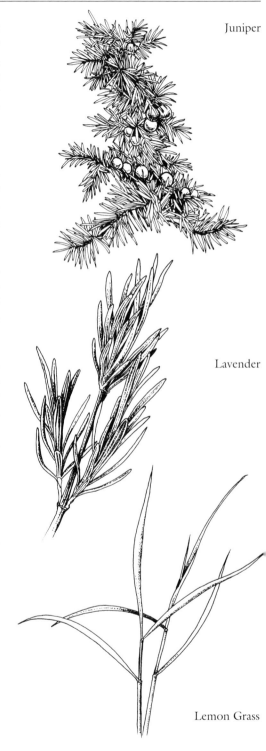

Juniper

Lavender

Lemon Grass

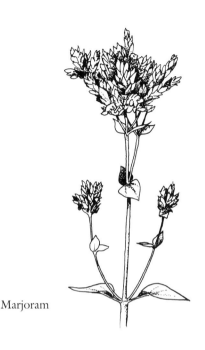

Marjoram

Myrtle Safe to use in therapeutic doses. Use on children over two.

Neroli This oil is safe to use on everyone including babies. Be careful if using outdoors in the summer because as it seems to attract bees, wasps and hornets, something that I have personally observed over many years.

Niaouli Safe to use on everyone in therapeutic doses.

Orange Increases photosensitivity, otherwise safe for everyone.

Palmarosa Safe to use in therapeutic doses.

Patchouli Safe to use in therapeutic doses. The smell is musty, musky and very intense and if adding to a blend you should use it more sparingly than other oils so that its smell does not overcome the blend.

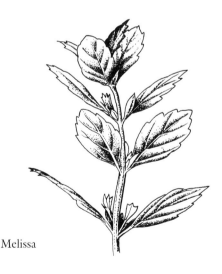

Melissa

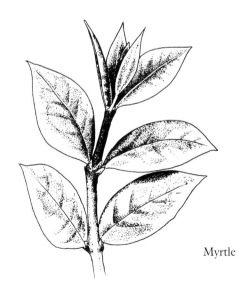

Myrtle

Peppermint This can cause skin irritation in some people while curing it in others. It is unsuitable for babies and children under fifteen, and should not be used by pregnant women as it is abortive. Spearmint is a milder form of mint and has been found to be less potent, so easier to use.

Petitgrain Non-toxic and safe to use on everyone in therapeutic doses.

Pine needles Safe to use in therapeutic doses. It can be used for children over two and is safe in pregnancy, although not if there is high blood pressure.

Rose Absolute All absolutes should only be used for their wondrous scent and the psychological benefits they provide. One drop is usually enough in a blend. Other absolute essential oils are: Jasmine, Violet, Gardenia, Mimosa, Carnation and so on.

Rose Distillation One of the least toxic oils, it is safe to use on everyone.

Rosemary Inhaling too much can cause nausea, dizziness and restlessness as it is a strong stimulant to the nervous system. Internal absorption can cause epilepsy and convulsions. It must be used only in low therapeutic doses and should not be used with hypertension.

Rosewood Non-toxic, safe to use in therapeutic doses.

Sage I have not included Sage oil in this book as my experience of the oil has been that it is very difficult to use, being fairly toxic. The smell is extremely invasive and has been found to make many people nauseous. It should not be used on epileptics, pregnant women, children and people with cardiac problems. Clary Sage has similar properties, but is less toxic so I tend to use it instead.

Sandalwood Safe to use on everyone in therapeutic doses.

Tea Tree Non-toxic; can be used on everyone in therapeutic doses.

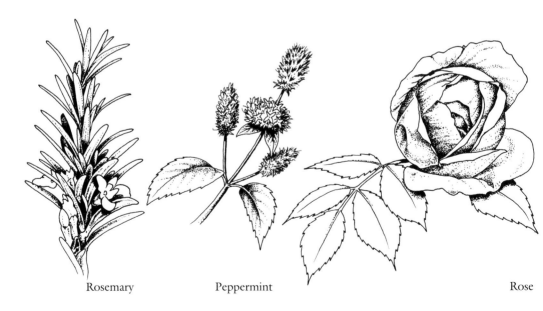

Rosemary   Peppermint   Rose

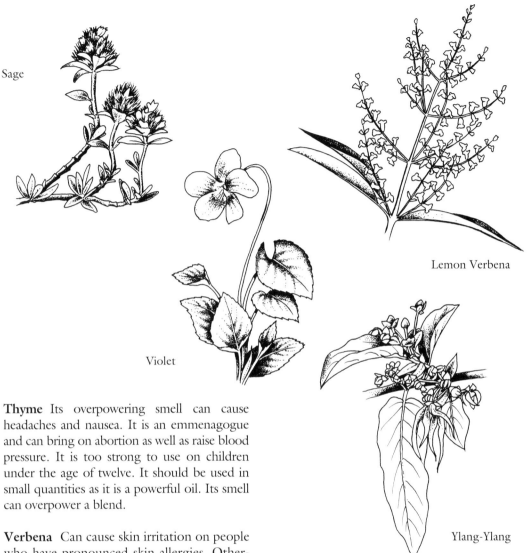

Sage

Lemon Verbena

Violet

Ylang-Ylang

Thyme Its overpowering smell can cause headaches and nausea. It is an emmenagogue and can bring on abortion as well as raise blood pressure. It is too strong to use on children under the age of twelve. It should be used in small quantities as it is a powerful oil. Its smell can overpower a blend.

Verbena Can cause skin irritation on people who have pronounced skin allergies. Otherwise, it can be used on most people, although it should not be used on babies or children under the age of five because of the potential for skin irritation.

Vetivert Non-toxic, but with a very penetrating, pungent smell and therefore should be used sparingly in a blend as it tends to overpower the other smells.

Violet Another absolute; use as with Rose or Jasmine.

Ylang-Ylang Inhaling strong doses can cause nausea, headaches, trembling and deplete the nervous system, so making you feel tired. Fine in therapeutic doses.

71

Current Generally Accepted List of Essential Oils Not to be Used in Aromatherapy	
Common Names	*Latin Names*
Almond (Bitter)	*Prunus amygdalus* var. *amara*
Boldo Leaf	*Prunus boldus*
Calamus	*Acorus calmus*
Camphor (Yellow)	*Cinnamomum camphora*
Camphor (Brown)	*Cinnamomum camphora*
Horseradish	*Cochleria armoraicia*
Jaborandi Leaf	*Pilocarpus jaborandi*
Mugwort (Armoise)	*Artemisia vulgaris*
Mustard	*Brassica nigra*
Pennyroyal (European)	*Mentha pulegium*
Pennyroyal (North American)	*Hedeoma pulegioides*
Rue	*Ruta graveolens*
Sassafras	*Sassafras albidum*
Sassafras (Brazilian)	*Ocotea cymbarum*
Savin	*Juniperus sabina*
Southernwood	*Artemisia abrotanum*
Tansy	*Tanacetum vulgare*
Thuya Plicata	*Thuya plicata*
Wintergreen	*Gaultheria procumbens*
Wormseed	*Chenopodium anthelminticum*
Wormwood	*Artemisia absinthium*

Essential Oils Not to be Used on Skin	
Common Names	*Latin Names*
Cassia	*Cinnamomum cassia*
Clove Bud	*Eugenia caryophyllata*
Clove Leaf	*Eugenia caryophyllata*
Clove Stem	*Eugenia caryophyllata*
Cinnamon Bark	*Cinnamomum zeylanicum*
Costus	*Sausserea lappa*
Elecampe	*Inula elenium*
Fennel (Bitter)	*Foeniculum vulgare*
Origanum	*Origanum vulgare*
Origanum (Spanish)	*Thymus capiatus*
Pine (Dwarf)	*Pinus pumilio*
Savory (Summer)	*Satureia hortensis*
Savory (Winter)	*Satureia montana*
Rue	*Ruta graveolens*
Sassafras	*Sassafras albidum*
Sassafras (Brazilian)	*Ocotea cymbarum*
Savin	*Juniperus sabina*
Southernwood	*Artemisia abrotanum*
Tansy	*Tanacetum vulgare*
Thuya (Cedarleaf)	*Thuya occidentalis*
Thuya Plicata	*Thuya plicata*
Wintergreen	*Gaultheria procumbens*
Wormseed	*Chenopodium anthelminticum*
Wormwood	*Artemisia absinthium*

CHAPTER 7
Therapeutic Guide to Essential Oils

Therapeutic Properties of Essential Oils			
Therapeutic Term	Definition	Related Essential Oils	Indicated for Ailments, Systems or Symptoms
Abortifacient	Can induce abortion.	N/A	N/A
Analeptic	Restores strength or stimulates certain organ functions.	**Aniseed, Coriander, Frankincense, Geranium, Ginger, Grapefruit, Lemon, Lemon Grass, Lime, Melissa, Pine, Rosemary, Rosewood, Thyme**	Good in the prevention of illness, in the convalescence phase and when the disorder is chronic e.g.: bronchitis – the lung tissue can be strengthened through baths and massages when the disease is not acute. The same applies to asthma, eczema, etc.
Analgesic	Can reduce, desensitize or stop the sensation of pain.	Camomile, Geranium, **Lavender,** Mandarin, **Marjoram, Melissa, Neroli,** Ylang-Ylang	Use for decreasing sensitivity or painful areas in the body, muscular aches and pain, superficial injury, cramps, neuralgia and skin inflammation.
Anaphrodisiac	Decreases sexual desire.	Essential oils which tend to act as natural tranquillizers, such as **Lavender, Marjoram, Vetivert, Ylang-Ylang**	Sexual obsessions and mental confusion.

Therapeutic Properties of Essential Oils *continued*			
Therapeutic Term	*Definition*	*Related Essential Oils*	*Indicated for Ailments, Systems or Symptoms*
Anti-arrhythmic	Abnormal or irregular heartbeat.	Angelica, Lavender, **Melissa, Neroli,** Rose	For palpitations caused by stress or after cardiac surgery. Check with medical authority before proceeding that it is appropriate.
Anti-bacterial	Destroys bacteria or inhibits their development.	Bergamot, **Cinnamon,** Cypress, **Eucalyptus, Ginger,** Niaouli, Palmarosa, Pine, **Tea Tree, Thyme**	Different bacteria need to be treated with different oils and it is not always clear at the outset which ones are going to be the most efficient. *See* guide to this table and ailments.
Antibiotic	Inhibits the reproduction of harmful micro-organisms in the body.	Cypress, **Eucalyptus,** Niaouli, Tea Tree, **Thyme**	These oils can be used on their own or while taking prescribed anti-biotics as they reinforce their action.
Anti-blotches	Remedy which prevents or diminishes blotches through vascular dilation.	**Benzoin, Geranium,** Mandarin, Myrtle, Rosewood	Blotches can be a reaction to certain products or after taking certain pharmaceutical remedies or due to age.
Anti-coagulant	Prevents clotting.	**Angelica,** Cinnamon, **Geranium, Neroli, Lemon,** Lime	These oils are either anti-coagulant or just help the blood to remain fluidic. The oils in bold are the anti-coagulants. They are needed when there is congestion of the circulatory system.
Anti-convulsive	Prevents convulsions.	Angelica, Lemon, Lemon Verbena, **Melissa, Marjoram, Neroli,** Rose, Ylang-Ylang	Can be used for hyperactive children or in an adult when there is hyperactivity of reflexes or even convulsions.

Therapeutic Term	Definition	Related Essential Oils	Indicated for Ailments, Systems or Symptoms
Anti-dandruff	Combats or reduces dandruff.	Camomile, **Cedarwood,** Coriander, Cypress, Lavender, **Rosemary** and Ylang-Ylang	Dandruff conditions can be brought under control by using a scalp rub.
Anti-depressant	Mood enhancer to fight depression.	Angelica, Bergamot, Camomile, **Clary Sage,** Citruses, Geranium, Lavender, Melissa, Rosewood, Violet, Vetivert	Depression often shows itself in the following symptoms: lack of stamina, sadness, lack of motivation, lack of interest in one's life.
Anti-emetic	Remedy which helps to prevent nausea or vomiting.	**Aniseed**, Camomile, Lemon, Lemon Verbena, Melissa, Orange, **Peppermint (in pregnancy use Spearmint)**	Nausea can occur in early pregnancy and can be difficult to overcome. One has to try one oil at a time to see what works. Travel sickness is another instance of nausea and sometimes when people are unwell.
Anti-histamine	Prevents or counters the effects of histamine in the body in cases of allergies.	Camomile, Geranium, Grapefruit, Lavender, Melissa, Mandarin, **Marjoram**, Petitgrain, Rose	Can occur in different parts of the body: respiratory allergies, skin allergies, digestive tract allergies.
Anti-inflammatory	Reduces inflammation.	**Benzoin, German and Roman Camomile, Geranium**, Melissa, **Neroli**, Niaouli, Rose, Rosewood, Tea Tree, Violet	There are different types of inflammation and often the essential oils that are good for skin are not necessarily the same when dealing with an internal part of the body or a joint.
Anti-migraine	Prevents or fights headache and migraine.	Camomile, Lavender, Melissa, **Peppermint**	There are different causes of migraine and various symptoms. Only the oils that are known to give quick relief of pain and tension have been included.

continued overleaf

75

Therapeutic Properties of Essential Oils *continued*			
Therapeutic Term	*Definition*	*Related Essential Oils*	*Indicated for Ailments, Systems or Symptoms*
Anti-mycotic	Destroys fungi and yeast or prevents their development.	Cedarwood, **Cypress, Eucalyptus, Lemon,** Myrrh, Palmarosa, Tea Tree, **Thyme**	Usually athlete's foot or ringworm and other unusual fungal infections contracted while travelling in tropical countries. These can be difficult to treat.
Anti-oedematous	Decreases accumulation of interstitial fluid under the skin.	Camomile, Cedarwood, **Cypress,** Geranium, Grapefruit, **Juniper,** Lavender, **Marjoram** and Rose	Relief of oedema will help proper reabsorption of fluid and encourages better healing in the body.
Anti-parasitic	Prevents or destroys invasion of parasites such as worms, mites, protozoa and others.	**Eucalyptus, Juniper,** Lemon, **Peppermint,** Tea Tree, **Thyme**	Only external parasites should be treated.
Anti-pruritic	Reduces itching sensations caused by the nerves.	Benzoin, Camomile, Cedarwood, **Geranium, Lavender,** Myrrh, **Patchouli, Peppermint,** Rosewood, Sandalwood	Any redness, itchiness, or blister-like rash can benefit from these oils.
Antiseptic	Destroys germs likely to cause infections or fights infections.	Most oils are antiseptic. First-aid oils for cuts and infected skin: Bergamot, Camomile, **Eucalyptus, Frankincense, Juniper,** Lavender and Tea Tree	An infection can cause the following symptoms: pain, redness, swelling and heat.
Anti-spasmodic	Relieves muscle spasm, muscular tension, nervous spasms and convulsions.	Camomile, Geranium, Ginger, **Fennel, Lavender,** Marjoram, **Peppermint, Rosemary, Ylang-Ylang**	Different anti-spasmodics are needed for different parts of the body. Some are better for muscle, others for respiration, others for digestion, etc. Look up the individual oils.

Therapeutic Term	Definition	Related Essential Oils	Indicated for Ailments, Systems or Symptoms
Anti-sudorific	Reduces perspiration.	Cypress, Lemon	Many people have sweaty hands and feet. There is no known cause of this problem but it could be due to nervousness.
Anti-tussive	Remedy which relieves coughs.	Benzoin, Camomile, **Cinnamon, Clary Sage, Frankincense**, Lavender, Mandarin, Myrtle, Neroli, Ylang-Ylang	Spasmodic coughs, particularly bronchitis-like coughs.
Anti-viral	Combat viral infections.	**Cinnamon, Eucalyptus Ginger, Lavender, Lemon, Lemon Grass, Myrtle, Niaouli, Pine, Tea Tree, Thyme**	Many of the essential oils are anti-viral and only the most common are named. They can help viral infection by using alone or alongside antibiotics.
Anti-wrinkles	Improves the appearance of the skin by toning down lines due to age.	Benzoin, **Frankincense**, Myrrh, Neroli, Palmarosa, Patchouli, Rosewood, Rose	Good when blending for face masks and moisturizers.
Aperitif	Stimulates hunger.	All the citruses are appetizers to various degrees, also **Aniseed**, Benzoin, Coriander, **Fennel**	These oils are useful when there is excessive weight loss as with anorexia.
Aphrodisiac	Increases sexual desire.	Cinnamon, Coriander, Ginger, Jasmine, Patchouli, Rosewood, Rose, **Ylang-Ylang**	Can be helpful where there is fear of intimacy, or sexual dysfunction, such as impotence or frigidity.
Astringent	Causes constriction of skin tissues locally.	Citruses are good astringents: Cypress, **Frankincense**, Geranium, Myrtle, Lavender, **Lemon Grass, Lemon Verbena**, Palmarosa, **Peppermint**, Pine, **Rosemary**, Rosewood, **Thyme**	Good to use on oily and spotty skin conditions. Mature and aging skin will also benefit.

continued overleaf

Therapeutic Term	Definition	Related Essential Oils	Indicated for Ailments, Systems or Symptoms
Therapeutic Properties of Essential Oils *continued*			
Balsamic	Aromatic substance from gums or resins, used to soothe the respiratory membranes or the skin.	Benzoin, Coriander, **Frankincense,** Geranium, **Juniper,** Myrrh, Patchouli	Useful when there is irritation and pain.
Cardio-tonic	Heart tonic which helps improve the function of the heart.	Angelica, Lemon, Melissa, Neroli, Rose	Very good after cardiac treatment or after chest infections.
Cardiovascular	Helps the function of heart and blood vessels.	**Cinnamon, Ginger, Juniper,** Lemon, **Marjoram, Peppermint, Rosemary, Thyme**	To improve circulation throughout the body.
Carminative	Frees the large intestines of gases and waste products.	**Cinnamon,** Coriander, **Fennel,** Ginger, **Lemon Grass,** Orange, Rosemary, **Thyme**	For painful flatulence, constipation and IBS.
Cephalic	Stimulates the brain or the mind.	**Aniseed, Basil, Frankincense,** Lavender	For headaches and migraines. Aids recovery from surgery.
Cholagogic	Stimulates the flow of bile.	Grapefruit, Lavender, Lime, Lemon, **Juniper, Rosemary**	These oils facilitate the early phase of digestion. Useful for indigestion or a 'hangover'.
Choleretic	Increases the production of bile.	Camomile, **Fennel**	As above.
Cicatrisant	Promotes healing of skin wounds and scar tissue.	Camomile, **Eucalyptus, Frankincense,** Geranium, Grapefruit, Lavender, Mandarin, Niaouli, Palmarosa, Patchouli, Rosewood, Rose, Tea Tree	Helps scars disappear.

Therapeutic Term	Definition	Related Essential Oils	Indicated for Ailments, Systems or Symptoms
Cytophylactic	Stimulates the production of new cells.	Bergamot, Benzoin, Camomile, **Frankincense**, Geranium, Lavender, Patchouli, Rosewood, **Thyme**	Important in the healing process of burns and wounds.
Decongestant	Helps relieve congestion.	Benzoin, Cedarwood, **Cinnamon, Eucalyptus, Fennel, Juniper,** Lavender, Niaouli, Tea Tree, **Thyme**	For sinusitis, colds, chest congestion, bronchitis.
Deodorant	Prevents odour.	**Bergamot**, Benzoin, Coriander, Cypress, Geranium, Lavender, Lemon, Lemon Verbena, **Peppermint**, Petitgrain, Rosewood, **Tea Tree**	Natural deodorants are useful in the summer for body odours and to keep fresh. They also help when people have to stay in bed at home or in hospital for long periods of time.
Detoxicant	Removes harmful toxins and metabolic waste products.	Fennel, Grapefruit, Ginger, **Juniper, Peppermint**, Pine, **Rosemary**	Recovery from illness affecting the liver, gall bladder or kidneys.
Digestive	Improves the work of the digestive system.	**Aniseed, Basil**, Bergamot, Coriander, **Fennel**, Lemon, Mandarin, **Marjoram**, Orange, **Rosemary, Thyme**	These oils are used for slow and painful digestion.
Diuretic	Stimulates the production of urine.	Bergamot, **Black Pepper**, Cedarwood, **Clary Sage**, Cypress, **Eucalyptus, Fennel, Juniper**, Lavender, Lime, Mandarin, Myrtle, Pine, **Rosemary**, Sandalwood, Tea Tree, **Thyme**	Diuretics are very important when trying to lose weight, treating colds and flu, and to detoxify the blood and restore stamina.

continued overleaf

Therapeutic Properties of Essential Oils *continued*		
Therapeutic Term Definition	*Related Essential Oils*	*Indicated for Ailments, Systems or Symptoms*
Emetic Causes vomiting.	It is not appropriate to use essential oils to induce vomiting but many of the anti-spasmodic oils can be useful for hiccups.	
Emmenagogue Induces or restores menstruation.	Angelica, **Aniseed, Basil, Cinnamon, Clary Sage**, Ginger, **Juniper, Lemon Grass, Peppermint, Rosemary, Thyme**	Useful for amenorrhoea and dysmenorrhoea.
Emollient Has a softening and soothing effect on the skin.	Camomile (German and Roman), Benzoin, Myrrh, Neroli, Palmarosa, Patchouli, Rose, Sandalwood	These oils are very useful for dry skin, scaly skin patches caused by eczema and psoriasis, and mature skin
Expectorant Helps removal of phlegm and catarrh.	Benzoin, Cedarwood, **Cinnamon**, Cypress, **Fennel, Frankincense**, Ginger, **Juniper**, Lavender, Myrtle, Niaouli, Pine, **Thyme**	This term applies first to the expulsion of mucus from the respiratory system but it can include the other excretory organs such as sweat glands, bladder and intestines.
Febrifuge Helps reduce fever.	Camomile, Cypress, Ginger, Lavender, Lemon, Orange, Sandalwood	The most important thing when dealing with fever is to cool it down if it is very high, and the use of cool compresses with one or two essential oils is very efficient.
Galactagogue Increased secretion of breastmilk.	It is difficult to use external application of essential oils to stimulate production of milk as the oils are likely to end up in the milk and be passed on to the baby.	N/A

Therapeutic Term	*Definition*	*Related Essential Oils*	*Indicated for Ailments, Systems or Symptoms*
Haemostatic	Stops bleeding and promotes clotting.	Benzoin, Camomile, Geranium, Lavender, Lemon, Rose	These oils are good for small cuts, profuse periods, and to help scar tissue to form after small surgery and in the case of bone fracture.
Hepatic	A tonic for the liver.	Camomile, **Fennel**, Grapefruit, Lemon, Lime, **Peppermint, Rosemary**	These oils are of great importance in convalescence, particularly after surgery for removal of the gall bladder and after hepatitis or jaundice.
Hypertensive	Raises blood pressure.	Ginger, **Peppermint, Rosemary, Thyme**	Very good for people with abnormally low blood pressure. These oils will increase high blood pressure and therefore must not be used when the condition already exists.
Hypnotic	Induces a state of trance.	**Clary Sage, Frankincense, Geranium**, Jasmine, Mandarin, Melissa, Neroli, Petitgrain, Patchouli, Rosewood, Ylang-Ylang	The hypnotic group of oils is very useful when there is acute anxiety, fear, and panic attacks. They tend to reduce hyperactivity of the reflexes and are good to use after shock or traumatic events.
Hypotensive	Lowers blood pressure.	Camomile, Lavender, Lemon, Marjoram, Melissa, Neroli, Petitgrain, Rose, Ylang-Ylang	These oils lower blood pressure and therefore should not be used when the condition already exists. Good to use for high blood pressure caused by stress.

continued overleaf

	Therapeutic Properties of Essential Oils *continued*		
Therapeutic Term	*Definition*	*Related Essential Oils*	*Indicated for Ailments, Systems or Symptoms*
Mucolytic	A remedy which helps expel mucus from the body.	Benzoin, **Black Pepper, Clary Sage, Cinnamon, Eucalyptus, Fennel**, Ginger, **Juniper**, Lavender, Myrtle, Niaouli, **Peppermint**, Pine, Rose, **Thyme**	Expels mucus from the upper respiratory passage during a cold, and with sinusitis and bronchitis.
Nervine	A nerve tonic.	Coriander, Grapefruit, Lemon, Lime, Mandarin, **Marjoram, Rosemary**	After recovering from stress, surgery, infections.
Parturient	Aids childbirth.	Angelica, **Clary Sage**, Lavender, Palmarosa, Rose	Many oils are not suitable for the labour room as they are so strong. It is important for the body to be relaxed while the mind of the mother is kept alert.
Rubefacient	Stimulates circulation locally.	**Cinnamon**, Ginger, **Black Pepper, Thyme**	Rubefacients are good for sprains and muscular aches.
Sedative	Calms, inducing sleep.	Camomile, Geranium, Lavender, Patchouli, Petitgrain, Mandarin, **Marjoram**, Melissa, Neroli, Ylang-Ylang	Sedatives help with insomnia, restless sleep and states of shock.
Stimulant	Increases activity and wakefulness.	**Basil, Eucalyptus, Fennel, Juniper, Peppermint, Rosemary**	Stimulants are stronger and more specific than tonics and are often needed after illness.

Therapeutic Term	Definition	Related Essential Oils	Indicated for Ailments, Systems or Symptoms
Stomachic	Tonifies the stomach.	Coriander, Grapefruit, **Fennel**, Lime, Mandarin, **Marjoram, Rosemary**	To help slow and painful digestion.
Sudorific	Promotes perspiration.	**Cinnamon, Eucalyptus, Ginger, Juniper, Niaouli, Rosemary, Peppermint, Tea Tree, Thyme**	When trying to lose weight it is important to have a good diet, exercise and a good excretory system. Also during or after illness these oils help recovery.
Tonic	Invigorates – either locally or generally.	Citruses are all very good tonics. Ginger, **Lemon Grass**, Lemon Verbena, **Rosemary**	There are nervous and cardiac tonics, general tonics and digestive tonics.
Topical	Remedy applied to the exterior of the body.	Many oils can be applied to the skin to help repair tissue damage.	N/A
Uterine	Causes constriction of blood vessels.	**Angelica**, Cypress, **Cinnamon, Fennel**, Geranium, Lavender, Lemon, Neroli, Myrrh, Ylang-Ylang	Can be useful after childbirth.
Vasoconstrictor	Causes constriction of blood vessels.	Cypress, **Juniper**, Lemon, Myrtle, Pine	Vasoconstrictors are useful in treating chilblains, and after childbirth.
Vasodilator	Causes dilation of the blood vessels.	Lavender, Mandarin, **Marjoram**, Melissa, Ylang-Ylang	Can help people who feel the cold, have poor circulation and when there is abnormally high blood pressure.

continued overleaf

Therapeutic Properties of Essential Oils *continued*		
Therapeutic Term Definition	*Related Essential Oils*	*Indicated for Ailments, Systems or Symptoms*
Vulnerary Helps the healing of internal or external wounds.	**German Camomile, Frankincense,** Geranium, Lavender, Palmarosa, Patchouli, Pine, Tea Tree, **Thyme**	Bone fractures and external and internal ulcers need vulnerary oils.

Note that the names of essential oils in bold indicate that these oils are more powerful in their activity than the others. Strength is not always what is required and the choice depends on the acuteness of the problems and their sensitivity.

Brief Explanation of Main Properties of Essential Oils	
Angelica	Remedy for deep stress and exhaustion. Recommended for grief and trauma and serious illnesses. Tonic for the nervous system; for cardiovascular system; for the lymphatic system and respiratory system. Mucus expectorant; digestive stimulant and anti-spasmodic.
Aniseed	Remedy for the digestive system; aperitif; nervous stimulant; cardio-stimulant; neuro-muscular stimulant; euphoric.
Basil	Central and peripheral nervous system and endocrine stimulant; digestive stimulant: particularly gastric secretions; excretory stimulant.
Benzoin	Respiratory system; pectoral, expectorant, anti-tussive; anti-inflammatory, cicatrisant for the skin. Suitable for children.
Bergamot	Endocrine regulator: hypothalamus and pituitary activity, nervous tonic and relaxant; skin antiseptic, anti-sebaceous, cicatrisant, anti-pruritic: shingles, cold sores, acne. Tonic of the digestive system.
Black Pepper	Circulatory stimulant, blood purifier; neuro-muscular tonic; digestive stimulant; expectorant; sudorific. *Note: can irritate mucous membranes and attack soft tissues.*
German Camomile (Blue)	Powerful anti-inflammatory remedy for acute skin conditions: psoriasis, weeping eczema, dermatitis.
Roman Camomile (Yellow)	Anti-inflammatory, antiseptic, analgesic, sedative, cicatrisant; febrifuge; slow and painful digestion; nervous relaxant and sedative; muscle relaxant: calms spasms and cramps; hepatic.
Cedarwood	Antiseptic; anti-infectious: vulnerary; respiratory decongestant, expectorant; lympho-tonic; anti-fungal.
Cinnamon	Sudorific, febrifuge; anti-viral, anti-infectious; neuro-muscular relaxant, anti-spasmodic; digestive system: constipation.
Clary Sage	Nervine tonic and powerful relaxant; stimulant of lymphatic system; stimulant of the reproductive system: emmenagogue, antiseptic; gynaecological problems; anti-sudorific.
Coriander	Tonic of the nervous system: relaxant and anti-depressant, stimulant: sensory system; stimulant of the digestive system: choleretic, carminative, aperitif.

continued overleaf

85

Brief Explanation of Main Properties of Essential Oils *continued*	
Cypress	Respiratory antiseptic, anti-tussic, pectoral, anti-spasmodic; vaso-constrictor, anti-sudorific, anti-fungal.
Eucalyptus	Respiratory stimulant and antiseptic, expectorant, febrifuge; diuretic, sudorific, anti-rheumatic.
Fennel	Powerful expectorant and mucolytic; diuretic, sudorific; stimulant of the digestive system: aperitif; antiseptic (mouth/throat); emmenagogue.
Frankincense	Respiratory antiseptic, expectorant; urinary system stimulant and antiseptic; nervous relaxant or stimulant; blood cleanser.
Geranium	Nervous tonic and relaxant, sedative, mood enhancer, endocrine regulator/stimulant (sympathetic hormones), haemostatic, tonic of the lymphatic system; anti-inflammatory, antiseptic, cicastrisant, vulnerary (fractures).
Ginger	Digestive stimulant; neuro-muscular relaxant; nervous tonic; blood cleanser, hypertensor; analgesic.
Grapefruit	Nervous tonic, digestive stimulant, mild diuretic, hepatic.
Jasmine	Psychological effects: uplifting to moods, beautifying.
Juniper	Stimulant of all excretory functions: detoxification; diuretic; mucolytic. Expectorant, blood cleanser; lympho-tonic: water retention; skin antiseptic and healing.
Lavender	Powerful tonic for nervous system: relaxant, sedative, anti-spasmodic; skin: cicatrisant, antiseptic, anti-inflammatory, anti-pruritic; tonic for respiratory, digestive and reproductive system.
Lemon	Gentle nervous tonic; digestive stimulant, hepatic; regulates cardiovascular system, hypotensor; gentle diuretic; anti-fungal, antiseptic; lympho-tonic; water retention.
Lemon Grass	Tonic, immune strengthener with digestive system (slow digestion); skin infections.
Lime	Antiseptic (skin and digestion), tonic.
Mandarin	Skin antiseptic; nervous relaxant and sedative, suitable for pregnancy and children; digestive, hepatic.

Marjoram	Nervous relaxant, sedative, anti-spasmodic; hypotensor; digestive tonic; stimulates repair for muscular and neuro-muscular tissues: sprains, bruises.
Melissa	Remedy for the hypersensitive: nervous relaxant, mood regulator, anti-depressant; anti-allergic; cardiovascular tonic; reproductive stimulant; digestive tonic: allergies, skin: cicatrisant, antiseptic, anti-inflammatory.
Myrrh	Nervous relaxant: anaesthetic, analgesic, sedative; skin: anti-inflammatory, antiseptic, anti-fungal, vulnerary, cicatrisant, anti-wrinkles; mucolytic.
Myrtle	Respiratory stimulant, tonic for nervous system; skin: antiseptic, astringent, anti-fungal; digestive stimulant.
Neroli	Nervous tonic and relaxant: anti-depressant, analgesic, anxyolitic, sedative; hypnotic: deep stress, trauma; mood regulator; reproductive system: menstrual cycle regulator; skin: healing, soothing, anti-pruritic, anti-inflammatory, antiseptic; tonic for the digestive system; cardiac regular: hypotensor.
Niaouli	Immuno-stimulant: pre- and post-surgery, antibiotic, infectious illnesses; tonic for circulatory system; skin: anti-fungal, anti-infectious.
Orange	Nervous relaxant: anti-depressant, anxyolitic, cardiac rhythm regulator, hypotensor; digestive stimulant: constipation.
Palmarosa	Nervous tonic and relaxant; skin: rehydratant, emollient, antiseptic, anti-allergic, anti-pruritic; lympho-tonic: oedema, water retention; regulator of the female reproductive system: mastitis, irregular cycle.
Patchouli	Nervous relaxant: hypnotic; skin: vulnerary and antiseptic (open wounds).
Peppermint	Powerful anti-spasmodic, analgesic expectorant, digestive tonic; (nausea); respiratory system: antiseptic and decongestant.
Petitgrain	Nerve relaxant: sedative (insomnia); skin antiseptic.
Pine	Respiratory and urinary antiseptic, antibiotic, diuretic; anti-arthritic.

continued overleaf

Brief Explanation of Main Properties of Essential Oils *continued*	
Rose	Cardio-regulator and tonic, nervous system relaxant: deep stress and anxiety, shocks, psychic unbalance due to deep grief, obsessions; reproductive tonic and regulator: gynaecological disorders.
Rosemary	Stimulant of the nervous system, cardiovascular stimulant: hypertensor, lymph drainage; diuretic; stimulant of the muscular system; digestive, tonic; skin antiseptic and astringent; emmenagogue.
Rosewood	Nervous relaxant, mood regulator; skin allergies: antiseptic; stimulant of the reproductive system and antiseptic: gynaecology and sexual functions.
Sandalwood	Urinary tract infections; skin tonic (oily, dry or aging), antiseptic; venous system.
Tea Tree	Powerful immuno-stimulant: antiseptic, anti-fungal, anti-viral; skin cicatrisant; diuretic, febrifuge, sudorific, expectorant, mucolytic.
Thyme	Powerful anti-infectious, anti-viral, anti-bacterial, antibiotic; circulatory and lympho-tonic: hypertensor; muscular relaxant; digestive cleanser.
Verbena	Strengthens the nervous system: relaxant, anxyolitic, tonic; deodorant, antiseptic; neuro-muscular relaxant.
Vetivert	Nervous system relaxant: anxyolitic; sedative: stress, insomnia; general skin care, insects and parasites.
Violet	Anti-depressant, calms emotional states, good for pessimism.
Ylang-Ylang	Nervous relaxant and sedative: shock and trauma; panic attacks; respiratory decongestant, expectorant; cardio-tonic and hypotensor; skin antiseptic.

The Essential Oils	
English Name	**ANGELICA**
Latin Name	*Angelica archangelica.*
Botanical Family	*Umbelliferae/Apiaceae*
Description of Plant	Angelica is a biannual plant that can grow up to 2m tall. It has characteristic wide indented leaves and large spherical flower heads. It also has a very distinct, penetrating odour.
Geographical Origin/Climate	It grows wild in Scandinavia, northern Europe and northern Asia. It likes wet soils with enough sunshine. Angelica is grown and eaten as a vegetable in Greenland.
Part Extracted for its Oil	Root.
Method of Extraction	Distillation.
Chemical Constituents	Main chemical constituents: terpenoid compounds: linalol, phellandrene, pinene. Sesquiterpenes: caryophyllene, limonene. Coumarins: angelicin, bergapten, umbelliprenin, imperatorin and angelic acid.
Toxicity/Potential Hazards	Abortive in high doses; photosensitivity.
Key Qualities	Forerunner of the stress remedies, a deep working oil.
Historical & Traditional Uses	It was one of the main ingredients in an elixir of life made in the Middle Ages; it was cultivated in monasteries of Central Europe and used as a remedy against the plague from the 15th Century onwards.
Medicinal Activities	The roots of Angelica are used widely in traditional Chinese medicine as a constitutional remedy in chronic illnesses. It is indicated for any disorders caused by deep stress and of psychosomatic origins. Angelica is one of the strengthening remedies where there is physical and psychic exhaustion. It is known to have a vasodilator effect on the coronary circulation and is strongly indicated for a 'weakened heart' and respiratory problems caused by vascular deficiency. It is also a tonic for the immune system as it acts as a preventive remedy with flu epidemics. Finally, it acts as a 'booster' to the immune and the endocrine system.
Contra-Indications	Low blood pressure, pregnancy and photosensitizing drugs.
Main Therapeutic Properties	For stress, restlessness and sleeplessness as it is: sedative, anxyolytic and hypnotic. Vascular deficiency: it is vasodilator and anti-coagulant. For respiratory inflammation, mucus, cough: expectorant, pectoral, vasodilator. For muscular pain, aches and spasms it is

continued overleaf

The Essential Oils *continued*	
	spasmolytic, anti-rheumatic, analgesic, anti-inflammatory. For poor appetite or slow digestion: aperitif, carminative, diuretic and depurative. For the treatment of dry, sensitive, delicate, damaged or infected skin: it is antiseptic, antibacterial and has anti-fungal properties. For painful periods: analgesic and spasmolytic.
English Name	**ANISEED**
Latin Name	*Illicium verum*
Botanical Family	*Illiciaceae*
Description of Plant	Star Anise is an evergreen tropical tree that grows to a height of about 4–5m. Its general aspect and its leaves look very much like Magnolia.
Geographical Origin/Climate	The tree grows in south-west China and north Vietnam. It prefers tropical habitats, particularly the rich soils of mountain slopes. It is cultivated in Japan and the Philippines.
Part Extracted for its Oil	Fruits.
Method of Extraction	Distillation.
Chemical Constituents	Main chemical constituents: 90% of anethole, safrol, estragole and eugenol. Terpenoid; monoterpenes: pinene, terpinene, linalol, limonene, phellandrene, dipentene, terpinolene, cineole; sesquiterpenes: caryophyllene, bisabolene, copaene, cadinene, farnesene.
Toxicity/Potential Hazards	Must be used in very small quantities. Excessive inhalation can induce euphoria, rapid heartbeat, light-headedness, headaches and muscular apathy.
Key Qualities	Aniseed induces a state of intoxication and euphoria.
Historical & Traditional Uses	Dioscoride always praised the sweet scent of aniseed to correct bad breath. Aniseed is part of the list of aromatic plants used in antiquity as a food and in medicine. It was first brought back to England from the Philippines by Thomas Cavendish. It is very much appreciated in aperitif drinks in France as Pernod; in Greece it's Ouzo and in Spain Anisette. Aniseed balls were a treat for children in Victorian days and are still a popular sweet in France.
Medicinal Activities	Star Anise is used to relieve the symptoms of digestive disorders: painful digestion, particularly stomach pain, slow digestion and flatulence. It is a powerful antiseptic of the digestive tract; it works wonders for halitosis, increases salivation and is a powerful appetite stimulant.

Contra-Indications	Pregnancy; hysterical tendencies and should not be used on children under ten.
Main Therapeutic Properties	It is a remedy for the digestive system and its main properties are: aperitif, digestive, anti-spasmodic, expectorant, stomachic and carminative. It has diuretic properties.
English Name	**BASIL (SWEET)**
Latin Name	*Ocimum basilicum*
Botanical Family	*Labiatae/lamiaceae*
Description of Plant	Basil is a plant that grows up to 1m high; it is easily recognizable by its heart-shaped leaves and clusters of small white flowers.
Geographical Origin/Climate	Said to originate from India, Basil spontaneously grows in the tropical and subtropical areas of the two hemispheres. In Europe, the plant is cultivated in large quantities in the warmth of the Mediterranean area, as well as being grown in greenhouses.
Parts Extracted for its Oil	Aerial tops and leaves.
Method of Extraction	Distillation.
Chemical Constituents	There are two chemotypes of Basil essential oil currently available. The first one has a higher content of linalol (up to 55%), while the second one has a higher content of estragole (up to 80%). Main chemical constituents: phenols: estragole, anethole, eugenol and safrole. Terpenoid compounds, monoterpenes: linalol, borneol, camphor, cineole, geraniol, ocimene, terpineol; sesquiterpenes: caryophyllene.
Toxicity/Potential Hazards	It is highly euphoric; excessive inhalation of Basil can cause headaches, nausea, followed by a feeling of disorientation. Can trigger fear and panic attacks.
Key Qualities	For the lethargic, it lifts the spirit.
Historical & Traditional Uses	The name 'Basil' is said to be related to the 'Basilisk', a mythical creature that could kill with a look. In India, Basil is the plant associated with Krishna and Vishnu, the 'giver and preserver of life'. Every Hindu house has a Basil plant to protect the spirit of the family. Protective in life and death, Basil leads believers to heaven. In France, has been used for medicinal purposes and purification, and in traditional Arab medicine Basil has been recommended as a cure for backwardness and cretinism.

continued overleaf

The Essential Oils *continued*	
Medicinal Activity	Basil is a powerful nervous stimulant, not to be underestimated in strength and it more particularly stimulates adrenaline release. Basil should only be used when tiredness is caused by a nervous disorder that slows down both the thinking and physiological processes in the body. More specifically it is indicated for halitosis, sluggish digestion; for muscular and neuro-motor problems; for M.E. and lymphatic problems.
Contra-Indications	Avoid using with epilepsy, convulsive conditions, acute stress, highly-strung states, pregnancy; it is not suitable for children.
Main Therapeutic Properties	Depression and despondency: anti-depressant and strong nervous stimulant. Anti-neuralgia: analgesic, anti-spasmodic, anti-inflammatory. Lympho-tonic, diaphoretic and diuretic. Stomachic, digestive and carminative.
English Name	**BENZOIN**
Latin Name	*Styrax benzoin*
Botanical Family	*Styraceae*
Description of Plant	This tree grows 10 to 20m high. Its trunk is rich in resin, but the tree itself does not smell of anything in particular.
Geographical Origin/Climate	Benzoin Styrax is a tree originally from Malaysia, Java, Sumatra and Borneo, found to grow at low altitude (200 to 500m), and near rivers. It is now mainly cultivated on the island of Sumatra in Indonesia.
Part Extracted for its Oil	Benzoin resin is collected from repeated incisions in the bark of the tree.
Method of Extraction	Alcohol is used to transform the resin into a liquid.
Chemical Constituents	Main chemical constituents: balsamic acids total over 20% – 9% benzoic acid and 14% cinnamic acid, 0.3% vanillin. Phenolic compounds mostly phenols; terpenoids: monoterpenes: coniferyl benzoate; 70% resinous compounds; ester: 2.3% cinnamyl benzoate.
Toxicity/Potential Hazards	Photosensitivity.
Key Qualities	Benzoin is the soothing balm to a troubled heart.
Historical & Traditional Uses	Benzoin was also called 'gum benjamin' by a famous Jewish Portuguese physician in the 16th Century. The word Styrax is derived from the Arabic name for the plant *asstyrax*. Benzoin Styrax appears in many recipes in Ancient Egypt and is mentioned by Ibn Batuta in the 14th Century. There

	is no reference of its uses in medicine in Europe until the 16th Century.
Medicinal Activity	Benzoin is very effective with itchy, inflamed, painful skin conditions. Psoriasis, abscesses, acne, dermatitis, shingles, urticaria, eczema, cracked nipples are all disorders which can benefit from the soothing and healing properties of Benzoin. Benzoin is often used to get rid of blemishes. It has been an active ingredient of many cough remedies because of its expectorant, anti-tussive, anti-spasmodic and soothing activity and it is very good for asthma sufferers as it is both efficient and gentle. It also has a pleasant smell and can be used as a deodorant.
Contra-Indications	Photosensitive.
Main Therapeutic Properties	General: Benzoin has antiseptic, anti-inflammatory, anti-wrinkle, anti-blemish, astringent, healing, soothing and vulnerary properties. Respiratory disorders: antiseptic, anti-inflammatory, anti-spasmodic, expectorant, anti-tussic, sedative. Good for children.
English Name	**BERGAMOT**
Latin Name	*Citrus aurantium* var. *bergamia*
Botanical Family	*Rutaceae*
Description of Plant	Bergamot is an evergreen shrub which grows 2 to 3m high with very fragrant white flowers. The fruits are slightly spherical in shape and are cultivated for their essence as they are not edible.
Geographical Origin/Climate	Bergamot trees are cultivated at about 200 or 300m above sea level, in Calabria, in southern Italy. Plantations extend from the sea to the foot of the mountains. It is also cultivated in the Ivory Coast, Africa.
Part Extracted for its Oil	The rind of the fruit.
Method of Extraction	Expression.
Chemical Constituents	Main chemical constituents – phenolic compounds: citroptenes, furocoumarins, bergaptene, bergamottin; terpenoids: monoterpenes: caphene, limonene, pellandrene, pinene, terpinene; sesquiterpenes: bisabolene, caryophellene – linalol, geraniol, nerol esters – 30 to 60% linalyl acetate; aldehydes: citrals.
Toxicity/Potential Hazards	Highly photosensitive, do not use when exposed to the sun or on sunbeds. It is phototoxic.

continued overleaf

The Essential Oils *continued*	
Key Qualities	Bergamot keeps us 'cool, calm and collected'.
Historical & Traditional Uses	Bergamot trees are said to be a lemon or lime grafted on a pear tree from Bergamo. The name of the fruit tree *bergamuti* is said to mean 'pear princess' in Turkish. In 1676, Paolo Feminis, a Calabrian, settled in Cologne and invented *Aqua admirabilis*; in 1818, it was sold to the rest of Europe as *Aqua di Colonia*. Bergamot leaves or the juice of the fruit were said to bring good fortune and prosperity to businesses and many people used to rub their banknotes on the open fruit as they believed that this ritual would force the notes to return to their owner.
Medicinal Activity	It is particularly indicated for infected skin conditions: shingles, cold sores, acne, athlete's foot and ringworm. It is refreshing and cooling as well as deodorant and is used in Eau de Cologne. As a nervous tonic, it is said to regulate functions connected to the hypothalamus, such as hunger, thirst, powerful emotions, moods and the hormonal cycle.
Contra-Indications	It is best to use diluted.
Main Therapeutic Properties	Bergamot essential oil is reputed for its fast-healing skin properties; it is antiseptic, anti-acne, anti-mycotic, anti-bacterial, rubefacient and deodorant. It is a nervous tonic, anti-depressant and has analgesic, sedative and anti-spasmodic properties. It also has digestive properties as it is carminative, depurative, diuretic and laxative.
English Name	**BLACK PEPPER**
Latin Name	*Piper nigrun*
Botanical Family	*Piperaceae*
Description of Plant	This is classified as a climbing perennial plant that produces green globular berries that turn yellow or red when they come to maturity. Black Pepper is harvested when it is just ripe. It is left to dry in the sun which makes it wither and turn black.
Geographical Origin/Climate	The Pepper plant is native to India and is extensively cultivated in tropical areas such as Indonesia, Malaysia, the Pacific islands and equatorial Africa. It needs plenty of shade and a very rainy climate.
Part Extracted for its Oil	The semi-ripe berries.
Method of Extraction	Distillation.

Chemical Constituents	Main chemical constituents: 70 to 80% monoterpenes: camphene, carene, linalol, myrcene, phellandrene, pinene, sabinene, limonene, thujene; 20 to 30% sesquiterpenes: caryophyllene, bisabolene, farnesene, elemene, bebene, copaene; oxygenated compounds: terpinene, nerolidol, pinone; 5 to 8% piperine, piperanine, piperettine, piperylline.
Toxicity/Potential Hazards	Can irritate mucous membranes and attack soft tissues.
Key Qualities	Black Pepper helps the shy and the timid.
Historical & Traditional Uses	The name Pepper comes from the Sanskrit *pilpali*. It has been used to strengthen magical talismans. To dream of Pepper was a sign of discordance and considered a bad omen.
Medicinal Activity	Black Pepper should only be used in small quantities because of its powerful inflammatory capacity. It should be avoided on people with eczema and varicose veins. In small quantities, Pepper stimulates digestive secretions and will speed the passage of food through the digestive tract. It can be used for sports massage, muscular pain and rheumatism. It has a stimulating effect on the mucous membranes and can therefore be used for chronic sinusitis. It is mildly sedative and stimulates the peripheral nervous system and is a very efficient treatment for nerve inflammation such as sciatica. Pepper moves the lymphatic system and is good for water retention and when there is a tendency to catch colds repeatedly.
Contra-Indications	Its use should be avoided on children's skin, during pregnancy, and when there is existing damage to skin, the blood vessels, or with high blood pressure.
Main Therapeutic Properties	Black Pepper is antiseptic, anti-bacterial, and has analgesic properties against neuralgia and pains. Pepper stimulates digestive secretions, it is aperitif, carminative and laxative. For muscular pains: it is anti-spasmodic, rubefacient, diuretic and sudorific. Black Pepper is a powerful expectorant, it stimulates the mucous membranes but can also irritate them.
English Name	**CAMOMILE (GERMAN)**
Latin Name	*Matricaria chamomilla* *Chamomilla recutita*
Botanical Family	*Compositae/Asteraceae*
Description of Plant	German Camomile is similar to the larger daisy, its petals are white with a small yellow centre.

continued overleaf

The Essential Oils *continued*	
Geographical Origin/Climate	German Camomile grows wild in southern and eastern Europe, but it is mostly the cultivated plants which are used for distillation. It is intensively farmed on the Hungarian salt plains and less so in England.
Part Extracted for its Oil	Flowering tops.
Method of Extraction	Distillation.
Chemical Constituents	Main chemical constituents: terpenoids: 25 to 50%; sesquiterpenes with matricine, proazulenes which give 5% of chamazulene when distilled; others: chamilline, ombelliferone; concentration of individual chemicals can vary from one distillation to another.
Toxicity/Potential Hazards	Possible photosensitizer due to the coumarins.
Key Qualities	For the delicate temperament of the English rose.
Historical & Traditional Uses	Camomile or *Chamaemelum* derives from the Greek *khamaimelon*, meaning earth-apple and *matricaria* comes from the Latin *matrix*, because of the plant's property to bring on the menses. The priests of Ancient Egypt dedicated the plant to the Sun.
Medicinal Activity	It is mostly used in Europe and the USA for its spasmolytic and anti-inflammatory properties. The oil is more appropriate for difficult skin conditions that won't heal such as: eczema (dry and weeping), urticaria, psoriasis, skin infections caused by fungi, allergies, dermatitis.
Contra-Indications	None.
Main Therapeutic Properties	German Camomile has antiseptic, anti-bacterial, anti-fungal properties; anti-inflammatory, healing, anti-allergy and vulnerary. It also has anti-spasmodic, calming, sedative and hypnotic properties.
English Name	**CAMOMILE (ROMAN)**
Latin Name	*Anthemis nobilis* *Chamaemelum nobile*
Botanical Family	*Compositae/Asteraceae*
Description of Plant	Roman Camomile is a perennial plant which grows to about 10 to 30cm high and has spindly stems and many soft hairy leaves of a lighter green than other Camomiles. It is very odorous. Hermaphrodite yellow flowers form part of its core. The yellow flowers are surrounded by a white ligulate female flower that forms the 'corolla'.

Geographical Origin/Climate	Camomile is native to European Atlantic climates and grows in many temperate places. It is cultivated in Spain, France, the south of England and many European countries
Part Extracted for its Oil	Flowering tops.
Method of Extraction	Distillation of the mature flowering tops.
Chemical Constituents	Main chemical constituents: terpenoids: terpenes: azulene and chamazulene; pinocarveol, anthemol; up to 75% esters: n-butyl angelate, isoamyl angelate, phenylpropyl; ketones: pinocarvone; coumarins.
Toxicity/Potential Hazards	Possible photosensitizers due to the presence of coumarins.
Key Qualities	For the 'eternal child'.
Historical & Traditional Uses	Camomile or *Chamaemelum* derives from the Greek *khamaimelon* meaning earth-apple and *matricaria* comes from the Latin *matrix*, because of the plant's property to bring on the menses. The priests of Ancient Egypt dedicated the plant to the Sun. Put some chamomile in your bath, it will kindle love. Camomile protects against spells and removes curses. There is a relationship between Camomile and the typical 'English Rose'. Roman Camomile is one of the remedies most suited for children and babies or delicate, sensitive people. It is useful not only when someone is suffering from particular ailments that require Camomile properties but also if the person is vulnerable, weak and 'burned out'. It is particularly indicated for PMT and PMS.
Medicinal Activity	It is good for insomnia, restlessness, hyperactive children and migraines. It can safely and efficiently be used for eczema, allergic reactions, dermatitis, infected cuts, abscesses, acne, blemishes. It is a digestive tonic, and can be used for hiccups, IBS, allergies, colics, digestive cramps. It can be used for bronchitis and asthma sufferers. It is also anti-rheumatic and anti-arthritic and can decrease pain caused by injury or arthritis to the joints. It is used for muscular and painful spasms.
Contra-Indications	None.
Main Therapeutic Properties	Camomile is antiseptic, anti-bacterial, anti-inflammatory, healing, regenerative, vulnerary. It is also said to be: anti-depressant, analgesic, sedative, calmative, anxiolytic and hypnotic. Digestive properties are anti-spasmodic, calmative, carmative, cholagogue.

The Essential Oils *continued*	
English Name	**CEDARWOOD**
Latin Name	*Cedrus atlantica*
Botanical Family	*Coniferales/Pinaceae*
Description of Plant	Cedar is a very tall tree, 30 to 40m high, whose spreading branches make it look like a large, irregular umbrella. It has blue-green long needles.
Geographical Origin/Climate	*Cedrus atlantica* grows in Morocco at an altitude of about 1,000 to 2,000m. The oil is mainly produced in Morocco. Some cedars grow in the Rif mountains in Algeria.
Part Extracted for its Oil	Wood and stumps.
Method of Extraction	Steam distillation of the ground pulp/sawdust.
Chemical Constituents	Main chemical constituents: terpenoid: monoterpenes: sabinene and sabinyl acetate; sesquiterpenes (50%): phellandrene, caryophyllene, cedrene, cedrol, altlantol, cedrenol, thuyopsene, cuparene, humachalene, atlantones.
Toxicity/Potential Hazards	Not suitable for children.
Key Qualities	Cedar is for those who live in the fast lane and need to slow down.
Historical & Traditional Uses	The word cedar comes from the Greek *kedros*. It was said to last beyond death because of its anti-decaying resins that can preserve the corpses of the dead. Cedar has purifying powers and chases bad dreams away. Burning its branches is said to bring prosperity.
Medicinal Activity	Cedar is indicated for infections of the respiratory tracts, particularly for chronic conditions, as its action is slow and its effects are more noticeable in the long term. It is known to be good for bronchitis and damaged lung tissue. As a lymphotonic, it can help lymph circulation, promote immune activity for the lungs and ease varicose veins. It can counter alopecia and can be used as a hair tonic. It has some healing property for the skin as it is soothing and anti-inflammatory.
Contra-Indications	Do not use during pregnancy and not on babies or children.
Main Therapeutic Properties	Cedar has antiseptic, astringent, anti-fungal, antipruritic and healing virtues. It has a preservative effect on the venous system, it is anti-haemorrhoidal, lymphotonic. Cedar is a powerful expectorant and diuretic and has emmenagogue properties. It is a sedative and relaxant.

English Name	**CINNAMON**
Latin Name	*Cinnamomum zeylanicum*
Botanical Family	*Lauraceae*
Description of Plant	Cinnamon is a tree which can grow up to 10 to 15m high. It has aromatic leaves which are oval and shiny. It has yellowish white flowers with an unpleasant smell and the fruit is a berry. The bark is used as a spice.
Geographical Origin/Climate	Cinnamon grew abundantly on Indian coasts. It is a tropical tree, growing to altitudes of about 500m, in sunny spots, especially in north-western India, Sri Lanka and South-East Asia. It is fond of alluvial soils. It is cultivated in Cinnamon Gardens (plantations).
Part Extracted for its Oil	Leaves.
Method of Extraction	Steam distillation.
Chemical Constituents	Main chemical constituents: phenolic compounds: phenols 4 to 10% eugenol, methyleugenol, eugenol acetate, safrole; terpenoids: monoterpenes: cinnamyl acetate, linalol, phellandrene, pinene; sesquiterpenes: caryophyllene, cinnamic aldehyde (65 to 75% of the essential oil), cuminaldehyde, benzyl benzoate; benzaldehyde.
Toxicity/Potential Hazards	Do not use in pregnancy as it is an emmenagogue and can start contractions and bleeding in pregnancy. Do not use Cinnamon bark oil.
Key Qualities	Cinnamon provides a 'fire' for those who procrastinate.
Historical & Traditional Uses	The word Cinnamon derives from the Latin *canna*. The Romans made wreaths with its leaves to adorn the temples of Venus, the goddess of love. A much valued spice in ancient times. The Dutch, who had purchased Ceylon and wanted the monopoly for the Cinnamon trade, bought from the King of Cochin part of the Malabar Coast and the right to harvest Cinnamon.
Medicinal Activity	It stimulates autonomic digestive processes. It is used for muscular cramps and when a part of the body has lost its range of movement, e.g. frozen shoulders. Excellent remedy for chest infections, congestion and flu; as it is very anti-infectious it protects against colds and flu. It is a warming oil and often is helpful when treating people who feel cold or who shiver at the slightest draught. This can be caused by poor circulation, low blood pressure or depression. It can help with extreme tiredness and can help to put on weight.

continued overleaf

The Essential Oils *continued*	
Contra-Indications	Do not use on children, on people with a sensitive skin, in pregnancy or with high blood pressure.
Main Therapeutic Properties	It is a tonic, sedative and a vasoconstrictor. It has many good digestive properties, more particularly it is anti-spasmodic, carminative and anti-bacterial. It is anti-infectious and anti-viral, anti-parasitic, sudorific; it is also antiseptic, astringent and anti-blotches.
English Name	CLARY SAGE
Latin Name	*Salvia sclarea*
Botanical Family	*Labiatae/Lamiaceae*
Description of Plant	This herbaceous biennial plant grows up to 0.80m high. Its leaves are very large, oval and hairy and its flowers are pink, mauve or blue-pink and grow in spiky, long clusters.
Geographical Origin/Climate	Clary Sage is found growing in the Mediterranean area, Central Europe and North Africa. Its favourite habitat is stony, arid ground, hillsides and on the edges of country lanes. It is cultivated for its oil in southern France, Yugoslavia and Russia.
Part Extracted for its Oil	Aerial parts.
Method of Extraction	Distillation.
Chemical Constituents	Main chemical constituents: terpenoids: 2.5%; monoterpenes: camphene, limonene, linalol, myrcene, pinene, terpinene; sesquiterpenes: caryophyllene, bisabolol, germacrene; sesquiterpenic alcohol: sclareol, terpineol geraniol, citronellol; esters: terpinyl acetate, citronellyl acetate, linalyl acetate.
Toxicity/Potential Hazards	Can cause drowsiness – be careful if client is driving home.
Key Qualities	Clary Sage stands for 'release' as it allows people to 'let go'.
Historical & Traditional Uses	The traditional name for sage is *salvia*, from the Latin *salvare* meaning to save, to cure. In the Middle Ages the plant was used to restore clear sight and it became known as *Salvia sclarea*, Clary Sage in English.
Medicinal Activity	Clary Sage is used a lot in aromatherapy to help with illnesses or problems with an underlying nervous cause. It is helpful to people who are uptight and are angry but cannot release their emotions; for states of high anxiety or fear. It tends to decrease hypersensitivity and the hyperactivity of many reflexes, it is therefore very good for bronchitis and asthma sufferers, eczema, dermatitis and psoriasis sufferers,

THERAPEUTIC GUIDE TO ESSENTIAL OILS

manic depression and migraine sufferers. It is also good for the hormonal/reproductive system, and has been successfully used with amenorrhoea, dysmenorrhoea, painful or profuse periods, puberty, PMS, menopause, ovarian cysts and endometriosis. It is also a muscular relaxant and anti-spasmodic and can be a healing factor in restoring joint mobility, particularly if there is paralysis. Good for depression, obcessive mental states, helps debility, mood swings, hysteria and tantrums.

Contra-Indications	Not suitable for children, pregnant women, or people with high blood pressure, mastitis or cancer.
Main Therapeutic Properties	Clary Sage has a strong affinity with the nervous system: it is anti-depressant, relaxant, a neuro-muscular regulator, anti-allergic, sedative. It is very good for gynaecological problems, is oestrogenic and an emmenagogue, and can help greatly with difficult labours. It is anti-spasmodic, anti-tussive and has some digestive properties. Clary Sage essential oil is renowned for its astringent, anti-perspirant, antiseptic and deodorant properties; it also has mild anti-bacterial power and is suitable for infected skin disorders.
English Name	**CORIANDER**
Latin Name	*Coriandrum sativum*
Botanical Family	*Umbelliferae/Apiaceae*
Description of Plant	Coriander is a perennial which grows to 0.70m high. The leaves at the bottom of the plant look like Parsley leaves but the upper part looks like Fennel. It has many tiny white flowers which give a small round fruit. The fruits contain the seeds of the plant; however, the fruits are often mistakenly called seeds. The fresh smell of the fruits is very different from the aromatic scent which develops once they are dry.
Geographical Origin/Climate	Coriander is an annual herb which grows readily in temperate and tropical regions such as the Middle East (Saharan oasis), northern India, South-east Asia, Mediterranean countries, and in some north European countries. Morocco, Spain, Russia and southern France are the main producers of the essential oil.
Part Extracted for its Oil	Fruits, seeds and leaves.
Method of Extraction	Distillation.
Chemical Constituents	Main chemical constituents: phenolic compounds: coumarins and furocoumarins; terpenoids: monoterpenes:

continued overleaf

	The Essential Oils *continued*
	limonene, pinene, terpinene; terpenic alcohols: borneol, 45 to 65% coriandrol, geraniol; esters: geranyl acetate.
Toxicity/Potential Hazards	Possible photosensitizer.
Key Qualities	Coriander increases integrity and sensuality.
Historical & Traditional Uses	Coriander comes from the Greek word *koris*, meaning a bug, named such because the fresh plant was said to smell of crushed bug. People used to burn a mixture of Fennel and Coriander seeds as incense to repel devils. In Ancient Egypt it was used as much in food as in medicine. Hippocrates praised its digestive virtues.
Medicinal Activity	Coriander is lighter than the other spices such as Black Pepper, Ginger and Cinnamon. Its warming and sensuous effect can help people reconnect with their body sensations after illness and trauma. It is recommended for extreme tiredness or weakness, dark moods, mood swings, bad temper and irritability. It is excellent for stomach ulcers, anorexia nervosa, colitis, constipation, IBS. Helps recovery from flu and colds. It is suitable for damaged, mature and dull skin and good to add to a natural aftershave because of its cicatrisant properties. It is said to help alopecia and its smell is liked by both men and women.
Contra-Indications	No known contra-indications and it appears suitable to use in pregnancy.
Main Therapeutic Properties	Coriander is a tonic, slightly euphoric, anti-depressant, anti-stress, anti-anxiety, analgesic and sedative. It is also an anti-spasmodic, but not as powerful as the other spices. It works a bit like Ginger on the digestive system but is more gentle and its effect is not so radical: it has aperitive, digestive, carminative, laxative, depurative and choleretic properties. It is also healing and anti-rheumatic. It can be used safely for the respiratory system as anti-bacterial, anti-fungal and an expectorant.
English Name	**CYPRESS**
Latin Name	*Cupressus sempervirens*
Botanical Family	*Coniferae/Cupressaceae*
Description of Plant	Cypress is a tall tree with a slender trunk, often growing up to 25m high. It has many ramified branches that give it its narrow pyramidal shape. Its leaves have a scaly triangular shape and the female flowers produce small roundish cones.

Geographical Origin/Climate	Coming from Asia Minor, Cypress is now widespread around the Mediterranean area and is often planted around cemeteries to act as a protecting wall. It is now very common in England as a decorative tree.
Part Extracted for its Oil	Leaves and young stems.
Method of Extraction	Distillation.
Chemical Constituents	Main chemical constituents: terpenoids: monoterpenes: pinene, sylvestrene, cedrene, cadinene; sesquiterpenic alcohol: cedrol and aldehydes furfural.
Toxicity/Potential Hazards	This oil should not be used for prolonged periods.
Key Qualities	Cypress stands for preservation.
Historical & Traditional Uses	The Latin name *Cupressus* derives from *Kuo* referring to a symmetrical box. *Sempervirens* means 'evergreen' in Latin. It is associated with Pluto, the god of the underworld. Cypress symbolizes magical powers that go beyond death. The wood was used to make the inner coffin to fit in the sarcophagus in Ancient Egypt probably because of the anti-vermin properties of its resin. Today, Cypress is often planted around cemeteries. Medicinally, it is mentioned by Hippocrates and later physicians as being very useful as an anti-pruritic and vasoconstrictor.
Medicinal Activity	Its anti-tussive and expectorant properties make it very helpful in stopping repeated, spasmodic dry coughs like a smoker's cough. It is used for bronchitis and chest congestions, both for its antiseptic and anti-spasmodic properties. It has antiseptic, astringent, anti-blotches and cicatrisant skin properties and can be used in cases of severe acne. Haemorrhoids and varicose veins can improve when Cypress is added to ointment and is applied externally to the affected area. It should be used in a cream form for 'heavy legs' caused by poor circulation and water retention. Its anti-sudorific properties are helpful for sweaty and 'smelly' feet. It is also an excellent remedy for athlete's foot and should be used with Tea Tree to reinforce the anti-fungal activity of these oils.
Contra-Indications	Not suitable for children under twelve, pregnancy and mastitis.
Main Therapeutic Properties	It is a neuro-tonic, is anti-infectious, anti-bacterial, anti-fungal, anti-parasitic. It helps the circulatory system: it is homeostatic, vasoconstrictor, venous and lympho-tonic, anti-ulcerative. It is a powerful expectorant, anti-tussive, anti-sudorific, anti-spasmodic, pectoral and diuretic.

THERAPEUTIC GUIDE TO ESSENTIAL OILS

The Essential Oils *continued*	
English Name	EUCALYPTUS
Latin Name	*Eucalyptus globulus*
Botanical Family	*Myrtaceae*
Description of Plant	This Eucalyptus tree is also called the blue gum tree and originates from Tasmania but there are about 700 different species of Eucalyptus trees. It has been imported to the Mediterranean area and North Africa where it grows on average to about 30m high; in Australia it grows to the greater height. The trunk is very smooth but its bark periodically peels off. The leaves are strongly odorous and balsamic, it has white flowers and its fruit has an angular shape.
Geographical Origin/Climate	The Eucalyptus grows wild in Australia, southern Europe and Asia. It is a fast-growing tree, very fond of water. It can reach very deep and draw water from the ground at the expense of other plants. It likes warm weather but survives very well in cold weather too. In Australia, it is called the 'fever tree' because of its febrifuge properties and its power in fighting malaria attacks. In Tasmania, it was used to drain swampy land, particularly malaria infested areas.
Part Extracted for its Oil	Fresh leaves.
Method of Extraction	Distillation.
Chemical Constituents	Main chemical constituents: monoterpenes: camphene, limonene, phellandrene, pinene, terpinene; citronellal, 70 to 85% cineole, carvone, pinocarvone, piperitone; sesquiterpenes: aromadendrene, alloaromadendrene, globulol, epiglobulol, ledol, viridiflorol, eudesmol; aldehydes: butyrald, valeriald, caproald.
Toxicity/Potential Hazards	Eucalyptus should be used very carefully and not for prolonged periods as it can cause kidney damage.
Key Qualities	For all the ills arising from stale water.
Historical & Traditional Uses	Eucalyptus derives from the Greek *eu*, meaning good or well, and *calypha* meaning covered, in allusion to the way the calyx covers the flower like a lid. Aborigines from central Australia used the berries for some of their rituals and associated it with recovery powers. Dolls filled with Eucalyptus leaves are placed on the bed of someone who is ill: the dolls laugh at the physician if the diagnosis is incorrect. It was used as a remedy against the plague in the 15th Century.
Medicinal Activity	It is the number-one remedy to fight many respiratory diseases. It will help fevers, flu, chest congestion, bronchitis

and broncho-pneumonia. It is used in cases of both minor or acute bronchial infections and for colds with a blocked nose. It calms down spasmodic coughs and in small quantities has a sedative effect. It can be used in vaporizations to prevent the spread of airborne infections. It is an ingredient in formulas to lose weight as it is a powerful diuretic. It is good for infected skin conditions such as dermatitis or eczema. As it is anti-fungal, it can be used against athlete's foot and ringworm. It is also efficient in the treatment of genito-urinary infections such as chronic cystitis, thrush and bladder infections. It should be used carefully as repeated use can dry the kidney tissue and cause lesions. It is also good for arthritic joints and rheumatism.

Contra-Indications	Should not be used on babies and children under ten years old, in pregnancy, with low blood pressure and photosensitizing drugs.
Main Therapeutic Properties	The Eucalyptus essential oil has anti-microbial, anti-viral, anti-bacterial, antiseptic, anti-fungal properties. It is a well-tried expectorant, febrifuge, anti-catarrhal, sudorific and pectoral. It is diuretic, rubefacient, a urinary antiseptic and is anti-diabetic.
English Name	**FENNEL**
Latin Name	*Foeniculum vulgare*
Botanical Family	*Umbelliferae/Apiaceae*
Description of Plant	This is a perennial plant which can grow up to 2m in height. It has finely indented leaves and tiny yellow flowers. Its fruit is oblong and pale green in colour.
Geographical Origin/Climate	Fennel comes from Persia but grows in western Europe, North Africa, the Middle East and western Asia; it is cultivated in France and America. The Fennel habitat is low altitude or near the seaside. It spontaneously grows on roadsides, cliffs and rocks.
Part Extracted for its Oil	Seeds.
Method of Extraction	Distillation.
Chemical Constituents	Main chemical constituents: phenolic compounds: 60 to 70% anethole, 5 to 20% estragole; terpenoids: monoterpenes: camphene, camphor, carene, fenchone, limonene, linalol, myrcene, ocimene, phellandrene, pinene, sabinene, terpinene.
Toxicity/Potential Hazards	CAUTION – can cause epileptic fits and convulsions on people susceptible to them.

continued overleaf

The Essential Oils *continued*	
Key Qualities	Fennel is the 'clear-out' oil as it helps the body get rid of wastes.
Historical & Traditional Uses	*Foeniculum* is the Latin name for hay. Should wild Fennel have spontaneously grown near your house, it is an excellent omen, meaning you live in an auspicious area. The essential oil of Fennel has been in use since the 16th Century.
Medicinal Activity	One of the best oils to use to lose excess weight and as a cleanser when trying to improve dietary habits and lifestyle. It is a good tonic to use in convalescence to prop up the system and increase stamina. Fennel is a very physical oil. It works particularly on the digestive system and improves the function of the liver as it is a cholagogue and choleretic, it has strong depurative and laxative qualities and is good for constipation. It also improves peristalsis. It is recommended for halitosis, gingivitis, tooth decay and throat infections. It is an emmenagogue and stimulates oestrogen and can be used for amenorrhoea and dysmenorrhoea.
Contra-Indications	Not for babies and children, or in pregnancy.
Main Therapeutic Properties	Fennel is a powerful diuretic, it is antiseptic for the mouth and throat. It is an expectorant and sudorific. It is also aperitive, stomachic, increases gastric secretions, is depurative, laxative, carminative and has galactagogue properties. It is anti-inflammatory as well as lympho-tonic and mildly cardio-tonic. Finally, Fennel is oestrogenic and an emmenagogue.
English Name	**FRANKINCENSE**
Latin Name	*Boswellia corterii*
Botanical Family	*Burseraceae*
Description of Plant	Incense from Africa is the gum resin of a shrub native to the desert regions of Arabia. It is cultivated and harvested by Somalis who cross the Arabian Gulf to sell it in the trading posts of Aden, Djibouti, Makulla and Zeilah.
Geographical Origin/Climate	This shrub has pubescent or tomentose terminal branches, composite leaves, white flowers packed in long, simple and erect clusters. The fruit is a drupe. The trunk contains deep canals which secrete a gummy, odorous oily resin if cut. This resin is what is used, the shape of 'tears' or 'chestnuts' (and refered to as soiled tears fallen on the ground).
Part Extracted for its Oil	Resin.

Method of Extraction	Distillation.
Chemical Constituents	Main chemical constituents: terpenoids: monoterpenes: cymene, myrcene, phellandrene, pinene, thujone, verbenone, terpenic alcohols: borneol, verbenol, varveol carveol; sesquiterpenes: caryophyllene, farnesol, humulene, cadinene, copaene.
Toxicity/Potential Hazards	Not for people receiving psychiatric care or on tranquillizers.
Key Qualities	Frankincense elevates the mind to the threshold of the spiritual world.
Historical & Traditional Uses	Frankincense was well known in Ancient Egypt and throughout the ancient world. Paintings dating back to the Queen of Sheba show Frankincense trees being carried on special litters all the way to Egypt where they were kept in boxes. People harvesting the resin had to be pure from sin as the plant represented the invisible bond between the souls of men and the supreme being. Frankincense is one of the 'sacred' perfumes and has been used by almost all religions for purification rituals and high magic to summon higher spirits. Ancient Egyptians dedicated it to the Sun and used it to purify the air at midday when coarser vapours from the Earth were drawn up from the deep, rendering the air hard to breathe.
Medicinal Activity	Frankincense is considered by many to be a spiritual oil and so use it for meditation. However, some find it too invasive and heady. Frankincense is a very healing oil for the respiratory system. It is recommended for broncho-pneumonia, to use alongside antibiotics or after the illness has receded as it tends to leave a vulnerability in the lung cavity. It is anti-tussive and can be used for repeated coughs caused by bronchitis or similar disorders. It is a pectoral, expectorant, bronchodilator and vasodilator. It is good for damaged, mature and aging skin and can heal ulcers and sores. It is anti-wrinkle and is used in regenerative face masks. It is indicated for despondency and loss of interest in one's circumstances.
Contra-Indications	Not an oil suitable for children or for people suffering from delusions.
Main Therapeutic Properties	Expectorant, urinary system, antiseptic for lungs, gums and skin, clears the head (of excessive fantasies), cleanser. The incense regulates sweat and is thus allotted anti-perspirant and deodorant activities. It also has antiseptic, astringent and rejuvenating properties.

The Essential Oils *continued*	
English Name	**GERANIUM**
Latin Name	*Pelargonium odorantissimum* var. *graveolens, roseum*
Botanical Family	*Geraniaceae*
Description of Plant	It is a shrubby evergreen perennial which generally grows to 1 to 1.5m. Its stems and leaves are very tender and break easily, and the leaves are hairy underneath because of the oil glands. It grows in clay or chalky soils.
Geographical Origin/Climate	It originates from the Cape of Good Hope in South Africa but the plants are intensively cultivated in northern Africa, southern France and around the Mediterranean area and Réunion Island. It prefers tropical and subtropical climates but is well adapted to temperate zones.
Part Extracted for its Oil	Leaves and aerial parts.
Method of Extraction	Distillation.
Chemical Constituents	Main chemical constituents: terpenoids: monoterpenes, phellandrene; sesquiterpenes: boubonene, cadinene, copaene, gayazulene; terpenic alcohols: linalol, citranellol, geraniol (75%), menthol; phenols: eugenol; esters: geranyl acetate, lynalyl acetate, citronnelyl acetate; aldehydes: neral, geranial, citronellal; ketones: bourbonanone, piperetone, mentone.
Toxicity/Potential Hazards	None, but should respect therapeutic doses.
Key Qualities	Geranium stands for equilibrium and harmony.
Historical & Traditional Uses	Pelargonium derives from the Greek *pelargos* meaning a stork. The first essential oil of geranium was extracted from the leaves of the plant, in France in 1819. Plantations in Algeria were first established around 1850 and the cultivation of scented geranium expanded into many warm countries around the globe. The most pleasant scent is extracted from *Pelargonium rosat* or *bourbon*.
Medicinal Activity	Geranium is indicated when too much stress is hindering the decision-making process. It also helps with acute shyness and anxiety. It helps severe depression, mental and physical debility, mood swings, irritation, stress. It should be used when there are ailments of psychosomatic origins. It is good for respiratory ailments such as asthma, bronchitis and respiratory allergies. It is good for skin disorders: dermatitis, shingles, urticaria, eczema, psoriasis; it heals ulcers, wounds, infected cuts. It is highly recommended to help the healing

	of bone fractures. It is haemostatic, and is good for varicose ulcers and varicose veins, and haemorrhoids. Its healing qualities are good for restoring tissues after childbirth and it is often used in the care of seriously ill patients.
Contra-Indications	None, but must be used in very small quantities and on children over five.
Main Therapeutic Properties	Nervous tonic, relaxant, sympathetic hormone regulator, homeostatic, lymphotonic, lymph decongestant, anti-inflammatory, antiseptic, cicatrisant, vulnerary. Major anti-depressant and anti-spasmodic.
English Name	**GINGER**
Latin Name	*Zingiber officinalis*
Botanical Family	*Zingiberaceae*
Description of Plant	Originally from India and tropical Asia, China and Java. Ginger is a herbaceous perennial plant that resembles a reed with an upright spiky stem and pale greenish flowers with purple markings. It has a fleshy, tuberous, aromatic rhizome from which the oil is extracted.
Geographical Origin/Climate	It grows in tropical monsoon climates; apart from India and China it also grows in Japan, Tahiti, the West Indies and Africa.
Part Extracted for its Oil	Rhizome.
Method of Extraction	Distillation.
Chemical Constituents	Main chemical constituents: terpenoids: monoterpenes: camphene, limonene, myrcene, phellandrene, pinene; sesquiterpenes: bisabolene, bisabolol, caryophyllene, sativene, camphene, copaene, ylangene, elemene, farnesene, zingiberene; (mono and sesqui) terpenic alcohols: nerolidol, elemol, citronellol, linalol, zingiberenol; aldheyde: citral.
Toxicity/Potential Hazards	Can cause dermal irritation on sensitive skin.
Key Qualities	Ginger fires up the mind and inflames the spirit.
Historical & Traditional Uses	The word ginger comes from the Sanskrit and is said to symbolize love and financial success. It is used for magic medicine by the inhabitants of a Pacific Ocean island where they chew the root and spit it on the sick as a cure. The same ritual is used to stop a rising tempest. Ginger has been in use for thousands of years in traditional Chinese and Indian medicine because of its preventive and curing

continued overleaf

The Essential Oils *continued*	
	properties. It is an ingredient of many Mediaeval recipes and was often used to induce an amorous mood.
Medicinal Activity	It is a great strengthening remedy, particularly suitable for convalescence after infectious and debilitating diseases. Ginger facilitates the passage of food through the gastro-intestinal tube. This can help people suffering from flatulence, slow and painful digestion, stomach ulcers, constipation and irregular bowel movements. Its aperative activity stimulates saliva and increases appetite. It is also recommended for the treatment of sprains, muscle tears, painful joints, rheumatism and sciatica. It is often added as an ingredient in sports massage creams.
Contra-Indications	Not suitable for children under twelve, pregnancy and high blood pressure, deep varicose veins and haemorrhoids.
Main Therapeutic Properties	It has tonic properties for all systems as it has anti-depressant, anti-spasmodic and analgesic properties. It is an anti-bacterial, anti-viral, anti-infectious remedy. It has many beneficial effects on digestive functions: aperitive, digestive, depurative, cholagogue and its activity keeps the liver healthy; it is laxative, carminative and a diuretic. It is a powerful expectorant as it is sudorific. It has anti-spasmodic, muscle warming, rubeficient, anti-arthritic and anti-neuralgic properties.
English Name	**GRAPEFRUIT**
Latin Name	*Citrus grandisi martinii* or *Citrus* var. *paradisii*
Botanical Family	*Rutaceae*
Description of Plant	The tree can reach 7m high. Its flowers are white, odorous and similar to but bigger than orange flowers. The fruit is usually spherical, pale yellow and it has a thick peel which is very bitter. The fruit is much larger than an orange.
Geographical Origin/Climate	It grows in tropical to temperate climates and originated from Asia. The fruit was not originally edible but was altered by culture with different varieties. It grows all over North and South America.
Part Extracted for its Oil	Rind.
Method of Extraction	Expression.
Chemical Constituents	Main chemical constituents: phenolic compounds: coumarins: limettin, meranzin and furocoumarins: bergaptene. Terpenoids: monoterpenes: 96 to 98% limonene; aldehydes: citronellal, geranial, neral, citral;

	esters: citronellyl, geranyl, beryl, perillyl, octyl acetate; sesquiterpenes: cadinene, paradisiol.
Toxicity/Potential Hazards	It is photosensitive and should not be used if lying in the sun or on a sunbed.
Key Qualities	Grapefruit is bitter/sweet and reflects the power to mediate.
Historical & Traditional Uses	Its Latin name, *Citrus paradisii* applies to an evergreen tree with fruits resembling lemons, *paradisii* from Paradise where it was found. It was considered very precious during long sea crossings at it can quench thirst and reduce anger.
Medicinal Activity	Its gentle tonic and regenerative properties makes it easy to use on children and adults alike. It is often used after surgery, particularly after the removal of the gall bladder. It cleanses the system without forcing anything. It is anti-infectious and can be used on very sick people and children who are poorly with other illnesses to fight ordinary infections such as a common cold. It can help lose weight and increase stamina.
Contra-Indications	Not to be used on sensitive skin as it can be a mild irritant.
Main Therapeutic Properties	Grapefruit is anti-inflammatory, anti-bacterial and anti-fungal. It is good for greasy skins and it has antiseptic as well as soothing properties. It is lympho-tonic and lympho-decon-gestant, a mild expectorant and choleretic. It is digestive and has choleretic properties, and is said to lower cholesterol.
English Name	JASMINE (Absolute)
Latin Name	*Jasmine grandiflorum*
Botanical Family	*Jasminaceae*
Description of Plant	Jasmine is a deciduous shrub with very odorous white flowers. Often climbing, it is an erect shrub, with dark green leaves and globular fruits the size of a berry. It grows in tropical and subtropical zones.
Geographical Origin/Climate	Jasmine originates from China and India, and is cultivated in countries around the Mediterranean area. It likes a lot of sun and the scent from its flowers is strongest at dawn. This is when the flowers have to be picked for the best smell.
Part Extracted for its Oil	Flowers.
Method of Extraction	Solvent extraction: absolute.
Chemical Constituents	Main chemical constituents: esters: linolyl acetate, benzyl acetate; terpenoids: monoterpenes: geraniol, linalol, sesquiterpenes: farnesol, indole, nerolidol, jasmone.

continued overleaf

The Essential Oils *continued*	
Toxicity/Potential Hazards	None.
Key Qualities	Jasmine stands for spiritual ecstasy and joy.
Historical & Traditional Uses	*Yasmin* is the Arabic name for Jasmine; the word may have derived from the Greek word *iasis* meaning joy. In India, brides put jasmine in their hair or wear it in garlands around their neck. It is a symbol of charm and is said to increase personal magnetism.
Medicinal Activity	The oil is obtained by solvent extraction and its action is limited to the psychological benefits triggered through the sense of smell. Jasmine is the oil that can beautify, and restore self-esteem and self-confidence. With this quality in mind, Jasmine is found to be exceptional for treating postnatal depression and nervous breakdown following alcohol and drug abuse. It is useful if women come to a point in their life where they feel like an unwanted 'battered flower'. For men, it is sensual and happy and refines the senses. Its scent has a sedative and analgesic effect.
Contra-Indications	None if used in therapeutic doses.
Main Therapeutic Properties	Psychological effects only are applicable – uplifting to moods, joyous, beautifying. Anti-depressant, astringent and cicatrisant.
English Name	**JUNIPER BERRY**
Latin Name	*Juniperus communis*
Botanical Family	*Cupressaceae*
Description of Plant	The Juniper tree is a conical-shaped shrub which grows 1 to 3m high. It is a slow-growing evergreen tree and its fruits are fleshy and round, bluish-green at first, turning blue-black.
Geographical Origin/Climate	Juniper grows on hillsides and in woods, it can adapt to any soil and is quite common in the northern hemisphere, Africa and America.
Part Extracted for its Oil	Berries.
Method of Extraction	Distillation.
Chemical Constituents	Main chemical constituents: coumarins; umbelliferone; terpenoids: 40 to 70% monoterpenes: cymene, geraniol, limonene, myrcene, pinene, sabinene; sesquiterpenes: humulene, cadinene, elemene; and many esters.
Toxicity/Potential Hazards	Stimulates thyroid activity, it is strong and should be used with caution. Prolonged use can cause kidney damage.

Key Qualities	Juniper cleanses and protects from malicious deeds.
Historical & Traditional Uses	*Juniperus* means acrid, and Virgil called it Juniper because of the acrid and sour taste of its berries. In Ancient Greece the smoke of its green branches was dedicated to the infernal gods and burning Juniper was believed to purify the air and chase away evil spirits. In central France Juniper was kept hanging on doors to repel snakes. Juniper berries give Gin its flavour.
Medicinal Activity	It can be used to cleanse a space or environment of airborne diseases like flu or when negative feelings seem to 'hang in the air' or atmosphere. Juniper is one of the best excretory 'body clearing' oils and can help people to become healthier and if needed to lose weight. As an expectorant Juniper powerfully expels mucous from the chest and upper respiratory passages. It is one of the best oils to combat mucous, coughs and bronchitis. It is a strong sudorific, antiseptic and diuretic, helping to ease elimination of water and uric acid and can be a great help when treating minor urinary infections. Juniper berry oil is recommended for osteoarthritis, rheumatic pains, gout and neuro-muscular affections (tendonitis). Given their carminative qualities Juniper berries are also recommended in cases of flatulence, colic and gastro-intestinal infections. It is a thyroid stimulant and the medical history should be looked at carefully before using Juniper oil.
Contra-Indications	Should be avoided in pregnancy, with serious kidney complaints or diabetes.
Main Therapeutic Properties	It is antiseptic, healing, astringent, regenerative and cicatrisant for the skin. It has anti-infectious, anti-bacterial, diuretic, depurative, anti-rheumatic, anti-arthritic, anti-parasitic, anti-perspirant, rubefacient qualities. It has expectorant, mucolytic, anti-tussive and anti-spasmodic properties. It is a powerful emmenagogue.
English Name	**LAVENDER**
Latin Name	*Lavendula officinalis*
Botanical Family	*Labiatae/Lamiaceae*
Description of Plant	It is a herbaceous plant which grows up to 60cm high. It has spiky stems that become woody after the plant is a few years old. The flowers are usually purplish-blue and come out in summer. It grows all over southern Europe.

continued overleaf

The Essential Oils *continued*	
Geographical Origin/Climate	Lavender grows freely in the Mediterranean area, specially on arid and chalky hillsides. It is cultivated in Europe and in the United States.
Part Extracted for its Oil	Flowering tops (aerial parts).
Method of Extraction	Distillation.
Chemical Constituents	Main chemical constituents: phenolic compounds: coumarin, umbelliferone, herniarin, santonin; terpenoids including: monoterpenes: 42 to 55% linalyl acetate, terpenyl acetate, geranyl acetate, lavandulyl acetate; camphene, carene, limonene, ocimene, pinenes, terpinene; gerania; geraniol, borneol, linalol, terpineol, lavendulol, cineole and linalol oxides; sesquiterpenes: caryophyllene, caryophyllene oxide, farnesene; aldehydes: cuminal, neral, myrtenal, lactones, benzaldehyde.
Toxicity/Potential Hazards	None in therapeutic quantities.
Key Qualities	Lavender mellows the mood.
Historical & Traditional Uses	Lavender oil and Lavender water were commonly used for their calming properties. Lavender has been used to relieve headaches and treat insomnia. Lavender is used a great deal in England and France. In the UK, until recently Yardley was the most famous English perfumer, with many products including the sweeter English Lavender.
Medicinal Activity	Lavender is used primarily for its anti-spasmodic and antiseptic properties, for First Aid and to calm down the person or parts of body system. Unsurprisingly for such a universally used oil, Lavender is used for many conditions. The list of the actions of Lavender is endless. Its high concentration of esters make Lavender an oil which works on the nervous system. Lavender is ideal for children and for a first time treatment. It traditionally reduces child and adult nervousness, notably in cases of sleep troubles. It is also traditionally used for mouth hygiene. Lavender is moreover recommended in certain respiratory affections such as asthma, crotchety cough, colds. It can furthermore be of help in cases of headache, spasm, flatulence, nausea and vomiting. Lavender also treats intestinal infections. Given its antiseptic properties, Lavender essential oil can be applied on infected wounds and burns. It is traditionally used to wash small sores and also to treat sunburn, superficial small burns and nappy rashes.

Contra-Indications	None in therapeutic doses, but the oil must be diluted well for asthma sufferers as it can create problems in some individuals.
Main Therapeutic Properties	It is an aperitif, carminative, cholegogue and digestive, excretory, depurative, sudorific and diuretic. Nervous system: it is a nervous tonic, sedative, analgesic, anti-depressant, a powerful anti-spasmodic for the muscular system, calms reflexes and is cardio-tonic. It is also antiseptic, anti-bacterial, anti-viral, anti-microbial, anti-inflammatory, cicatrisant, vulnerary and healing. It is an amazing healer of skin burns, and is also anti-tussive, decongestant, mucolytic and a general spasmolytic.
English Name	**LEMON**
Latin Name	*Citrus limonum*
Botanical Family	*Rutaceae*
Description of Plant	It is a small evergreen tree which grows 3 to 5m high and is very similar to an Orange tree.
Geographical Origin/Climate	Coming orginally from India, the Lemon tree is now also grown in California and in the Mediterranean area.
Part Extracted for its Oil	Rind.
Method of Extraction	Expression.
Chemical Constituents	Main chemical constituents: phenolic compounds; coumarins, umbelliferone, scopoletin and furocoumarins bergaptene, bergamottin, bergaptol, citroptene; terpenoids: mono-terpenes: geranyl acetate, linalyl acetate, 55 to 80% limonene, terpinene, terpineolene; sesquiterpenes: bisabolene; aliphatic alcohols: hexanol, octanol, nonanol, decanol. Aldehydes: citral, geranial, hexanal, heptanal, octanal, nonanal.
Toxicity/Potential Hazards	Phototoxicity, photosensitivity.
Key Qualities	Lemon brings the zest of life.
Historical & Traditional Uses	The name Lemon derives from *lima* which means Small Lemon in Arabic. People used to use Lemon juice to cleanse and disinfect as it was known to purify. In Mid-America women baked Lemon tarts to prevent conjugal infidelity.
Medicinal Activity	All citrus oils are 'user friendly' – great for first treatments, beneficial where they act on the nervous system, and are a tonic for the body. They act quickly, their actions are beneficial but short lived and are agreeable to all. Lemon is

continued overleaf

The Essential Oils *continued*	
	good for the whole digestion, it aids the appetite, helps purify the liver and the blood and regulates bile secretion. It is a nervous tonic, helps with depression, lack of stamina and tiredness. For the cardiovascular systems, it is particularly good for varicose veins and capillarial circulation. It circulates the lymph and helps with obesity. It is a mild decongestant and can be used for children (mixed with Benzoin) for chest infections. It is one of the best oils against arthritis, rheumatism and gout.
Contra-Indications	This oil is highly photosensitive and can irritate children's skin and should therefore be used sparingly and well diluted on sensitive skins.
Main Therapeutic Properties	Lemon is a nervous tonic and an anti-depressant, anti-infectious, anti-bacterial, anti-fungal, antiseptic, astringent, rubefacient and has a regulating effect. It is also a tonic for the cardiovascular system; it regulates blood pressure, and has lympho-tonic, diuretic, stomachic, hepatic and digestive properties. It is good for oily skin, acne and warts.
English Name	**LEMON GRASS**
Latin Name	*Cymbopogon citratus*
Botanical Family	*Gramineae*
Description of Plant	Lemon Grass is not to be confused with Lemon Verbena or Lemon Balm (Melissa), both growing in northern latitudes. It is cultivated in the warm areas of Asia and China, Africa and America. This is a grass which can grow up to half a metre high and has vibrant green, ribbon-shaped leaves. It produces numerous blue/purple flowers.
Geographical Origin/Climate	It originates from the southern part of India in Madras where it grows wild, but most of the oil production comes from Travancore and Nellampatty in the state of Cochin. This plant needs a lot of warmth and water to grow fully and it prefers the natural 'greenhouse' of the planet (monsoon regions) as a habitat. It grows freely in many hot countries and is also widely cultivated. It is found in Africa, Madagascar, Sri Lanka, Java, Malaysia and the West Indies.
Part Extracted for its Oil	Leaves and aerial parts.
Method of Extraction	Distillation.
Chemical Constituents	Main chemical constituents: terpenoids: monoterpenes: citronellal, citronellol, geraniol, linalol, 12 to 20% myrcene, terpinol, nerol; aldehydes: 65 to 80% citral, geranial,

farnesal, cymbopogonol; sesquiterpenes: farnesol.

Toxicity/Potential Hazards	Can cause major skin irritation on those with sensitive skin.
Key Qualities	Lemon Grass invites sensory excitement.
Historical & Traditional Uses	The plant has been cultivated in India for a very long time, more particularly in south-west India. It has been used as a febrifuge and for many local infectious illnesses. The oil is a little bit different and is more suitable for digestive ailments.
Medicinal Activity	Lemon Grass is good for problems of the muscular and the digestive system if caused by poor abdominal muscle tone or obesity. It is helpful for indigestion, stomach pains due to slow digestion, hiatus hernia, heartburn and flatulence. It is a tonic to the nervous system, and helps people who lack confidence. However, it is not suitable for everyone and it should be used sparingly as it is fairly strong.
Contra-Indications	Avoid in pregnancy, and not for children who are eczema sufferers.
Main Therapeutic Properties	It has vermifuge, anti-parasitic, anti-bacterial and anti-fungal properties. It is mildly analgesic, anti-spasmodic, sudorific, diuretic, digestive and an emmenagogue. It is also astringent, regulates sebaceous secretion and is a digestive and skin antiseptic.
English Name	LIME
Latin Name	*Citrus limetta*
Botanical Family	*Rutaceae*
Description of Plant	The Lime tree is one of the citrus trees and its branches and leaves are very similar to the Lemon and Orange trees. It produces white flowers and its fruit is smaller than a lemon and is green in colour, although with age it will turn yellow-green. The skin is very bitter.
Geographical Origin/Climate	The Lime tree is indigenous to India, but most of the cultivation takes place around Bombay. It is cultivated in many countries such as Florida, Mexico, Jamaica, Africa.
Part Extracted for its Oil	Rind.
Method of Extraction	Expression.
Chemical Constituents	Main chemical constituents: terpenoids: monoterpernes: limonene, (50 to 70%), citral, linalyl acetate, terpinenes, cymene; alcohols: linalol coumarins: auraptene, bergamotin, angelicin, limettin.

continued overleaf

The Essential Oils *continued*	
Toxicity/Potential Hazards	Highly photosensitive.
Key Qualities	Lime is the revitalizing remedy.
Historical & Traditional Uses	Used as an aperitif, digestive and depurative of the digestive system, it is served in India and other countries with water to quench thirst. It has many similar properties to Lemon and Bergamot.
Medicinal Activity	Lime is good for oily and spotty skins; it helps the liver to do its work and generally stimulates gastric juices and facilitates excretion of food wastes.
Contra-Indications	Another photosensitive oil and can be slightly irritant to children's or sensitive skins.
Main Therapeutic Properties	Antiseptic (skin and digestion), deodorant, aperitive, hepatic, anti-bacterial, depurative; it is a great tonic and a refreshing oil.
English Name	**MANDARIN**
Latin Name	*Citrus reticulata*
Botanical Family	*Rutaceae*
Description of Plant	The Mandarin shrub/tree grows to 5 to 8m high, it has many branches, a dense foliage with oblong and slightly tough leaves; it bears small white flowers. The fruit is bright orange and the essential oil sacks are very visible on the surface of the rind, with small depressions which contain the essence.
Geographical Origin/Climate	The Mandarin tree is native to Asia, particularly China and Japan. It was imported from Indo-China into the western part of the Mediterranean area in 1828. The main producers today are Sicily, Greece, Brazil, USA.
Part Extracted for its Oil	Rind.
Method of Extraction	Expression.
Chemical Constituents	Main chemical constituents: contains a number of coumarins, furocoumarins; terpenoids: monoterpenes (65 to 75%) limonene, terpinene, pinene; ester: benzyle acetate; alcohols: citronellol, geraniol, linalol aldehydes: citral, citronellal.
Toxicity/Potential Hazards	Photosensitivity.
Key Qualities	Mandarin is for easy relaxing.
Historical & Traditional Uses	The Mandarin originates from the Chinese and is a symbol of good fortune. As a gift it was obviously fit to be given to a Mandarin and it is still a traditional gift in China, where it

	is given at lunar celebrations.
Medicinal Activity	Mandarin is a light, mildly hypnotic and sedative oil which helps the restless mind to sleep. It can be used safely for pregnant women, babies (diluted), children and everyone. Its aroma is reminiscent of sweets and many children find Mandarin very agreeable. It helps digestion and is good for stomach ulcers, and any spasmodic digestive problems. As it decreases the hyper-activity of the digestive system it is also good for allergies, colics, hiccups etc. It can help with losing weight and is recommended for people in poor health who are obese or for cellulite. For the skin, it can be added to a steam facial as it is a good, gentle cleanser.
Contra-Indications	Photosensitivity.
Main Therapeutic Properties	It is a tonic, analgesic, anti-spasmodic, sedative and stimulates para-sympathetic activity. It is cholagogue, digestive, carminative, diuretic and laxative. It stimulates lymphatic circulation and has anti-oedematous properties. It is also antiseptic, anti-bacterial and anti-fungal.
English Name	**(SWEET) MARJORAM**
Latin Name	*Origanum marjorana*
Botanical Family	*Labiateae/Lamiaceae*
Description of Plant	A perennial plant which grows 20 to 50cm in height and tends to propagate very efficiently. It usually has small, oval and velvety leaves, yellow-green on the top and greyish underneath. Its very tiny whitish or pinkish flowers give out a very aromatic smell. Marjoram is often confused with oregano.
Geographical Origin/Climate	Likes to grow in sunny places in the Mediterranean area and North Africa where it is cultivated, particularly in Tunisia. Also cultivated in India, Egypt and Arabia.
Part Extracted for its Oil	Flowering tops/leaf.
Method of Extraction	Distillation.
Chemical Constituents	Main chemical constituents: phenolic compounds: phenols, anethole, eugenol, estragole and carvacrol; terpenoids: monoterpenes: esters: linalyl acetate, terpenyl acetate, geranyl acetate, linalol, myrcene, phellandrenes, pinene, sabinene, terpinene, terpineol, terpineolene, cymene, thujanol and ocimene; sesquiterpenes: caryophyllene.
Toxicity/Potential Hazards	Causes disorientation and mild apathy if used over the therapeutic dosage.

continued overleaf

The Essential Oils *continued*	
Key Qualities	Marjoram dissipates inner torment.
Historical & Traditional Uses	Marjoram possibly derives from the Latin word for 'bigger' or Marjory, the French Provençale for the name of the Virgin Mary. *Origanum* means 'beauty', a reference to the beautiful habitat in which Marjoram plants can be found. It was used in Ancient Egypt, Greece and Italy as an aromatic for food and a well-respected medicinal plant. In Ancient Greece it had an affinity with the dead as Marjoram was planted on tombs to ensure that the dead rested in peace. Marjoram was also said to drive seducers away.
Medicinal Activity	Marjoram is said to strengthen the nervous system. The oil acts as a very powerful anxiolitic and sedative and is good for stress. It is often used for insomnia and for people who are 'highly strung' and over wilful. It also suits people who always make rash decisions and find it difficult to think and concentrate. It calms the mind and as with all anaphrodisiacs will decrease sexual obsessions. It can be used for epileptics; it calms down thyroid activity and can be used for people who have 'borderline' hyperthyroid symptoms. It is a hypotensor and works well for high blood pressure sufferers. It calms down palpitations, particularly if stemming from stress. It is very good to clear the body of mucous and can calm down spasmodic coughs; it is a broncho-dilator and is excellent for bronchitis, asthma, flu, whooping cough and ordinary coughs. It is an antiseptic and anti-spasmodic of the digestive system: it will calm down excessive hydrochloric acid secretions; it is good for the treatment of ulcers, colitis and hiccups; it stimulates digestion and is carminative and good for mouth hygiene. For the skin it is antiseptic and is said to help depigmentation as well as lighten up the skin. However, as it is strong use only in the therapeutic dosage.
Contra-Indications	This is a strong sedative and can cause drowsiness. If adding to a blend, use more sparingly than other oils. Not suitable for children, babies and early pregnancy.
Main Therapeutic Properties	It is sedative, slows down reflexes, anaphrodisiac. It has digestive, aperitive, laxative, carminative, sudorific and stimulant properties. It is also expectorant, diuretic, anti-oedematous, broncho-dilator, anti-rheumatism, anti-migraine, anti-virus. It is vasodilating, hypotensive and emmenagogue. Finally, it has anti-bacterial and anti-fungal properties.

English Name	**MELISSA**
Latin Name	*Melissa officinalis*
Botanical Family	*Labiateae/Lamiaceae*
Description of Plant	Melissa is a traditional herb that can be found in most herb gardens. It has green or yellowish leaves similar to nettles but a little bit rounder and much softer. It bears white flowers with a mauve tinge and has a very strong lemony smell.
Geographical Origin/Climate	Melissa grows in many places, both wild and cultivated. Originally from temperate warm zones like most *Labiateae* it is also cultivated in North Africa, North America, in the Middle East and Europe.
Part Extracted for its Oil	Stems/Leaf.
Method of Extraction	Distillation. This oil is often adulterated.
Chemical Constituents	Main chemical constituents: phenolic compounds: eugenol; terpenoids: monoterpenes: citronellol, geraniol, ocimene, aldehyde: citral, neral; geranial, citronellal; esters: neryl acetate, citronnellyl, geranyl acetate; sesquiterpenes: caryophyllene.
Toxicity/Potential Hazards	None when used in therapeutic doses.
Key Qualities	Melissa is the remedy for melancholy.
Historical & Traditional Uses	Melissa is a plant that was known well to the ancient Greek, Roman and Arab physicians. Theophrastus called Melissa 'melissophyllon' and gave it vulnerary and sedative properties. The Arabs believed that it removed all anxiety, fears and melancholic humours. It has the long-standing reputation of gladdening the heart and curing hypochondria.
Medicinal Activity	Melissa is one of the traditional remedies for sadness, nervousness and anxiety. It suits both adults and children and can be used in cases of minor sleep troubles, psychosomatic problems, particularly pain with no obvious cause behind it such as 'tummy ache' or headaches; painful digestion, muscular aches, painful periods. Melissa has a soothing and sedative activity and is good for treating people suffering from panic attacks, palpitations, fearful states and hysteria. It is also ideal for people who live in fear of being seriously ill. For them, Melissa is known to be a natural tranquillizer, with hypnotic properties. It can help oversensitive people in general but also the ones who suffer

continued overleaf

121

The Essential Oils *continued*	
	from mental illness, as it can calm down fears. It is recommended for hysteria, delirium, delusions, excessive fantasies, chronic depression and despondency. It is often used for grief when the grief is connected to the loss of a child. Melissa can also be used to treat travel sickness or nausea.
Contra-Indications	Safe to use on everyone in therapeutic doses.
Main Therapeutic Properties	Melissa is antiseptic, anti-bacterial, anti-viral, anti-inflammatory, anti-allergy, cicatrisant and healing. It has digestive, choleretic, diuretic, depurative, carminative and sudorific properties. It is sedative, tranquillizing, anti-spasmodic and anti-histamine.
English Name	**MYRRH**
Latin Name	*Commiphora molmol* *Commiphora abyssinica, Commiphora myrrha*
Botanical Family	*Burseraceae*
Description of Plant	The Myrrh shrub grows to roughly 10m high. Its leaves are strongly aromatic and it has secretory canals located under the bark. Myrrh gum is a thick dark liquid which exudes from the natural cracks of the thin bark. The inhabitants of Somalia and the Yemen harvest the gum by making several incisions in the tree. When the gum comes out as a liquid it then solidifies and looks like whitish tears. When it dries it turns reddish.
Geographical Origin/Climate	Myrrh is a thorny tree native to the arid areas of western Africa. It was imported to grow in Egypt a long time ago; it also grows in Arabia, Ethiopia, the Sudan and Somalia.
Part Extracted for its Oil	Gum/Resin.
Method of Extraction	Distillation of the gum.
Chemical Constituents	Main chemical constituents: phenolic compounds: phenols: eugenol; terpenoids: monoterpenes such as limonene, pinene, copaene, isolinalyl acetate; aldehydes: cuminic aldehyde and cinnamic aldehyde.
Toxicity/Potential Hazards	None.
Key Qualities	Myrrh protects from full moon madness.
Historical & Traditional Uses	The word Myrrh originates from the Greek word *Myrrha*, which means fragrant. Myrrh is mentioned in many religious scriptures from a great number of civilizations. It

	has been used for rituals, for cleansing by fumigation and the Ancient Egyptians believed that its smell protected from dark influences. The New Testament makes many references to Myrrh and its merits are countless as it is used as a perfume, incense or for medicinal purposes. Distillation of the essential oil was already known in the 16th Century.
Medicinal Activity	With its highly anaesthetic, antiseptic aroma, reminiscent of the dental surgery, Myrrh has an age-old tradition of uses in ritual and in medicine and its very earthy smell is very grounding. It can be worn as a perfume to dispel dark influences, and offer protection during a difficult time in life (serious illness). Its anti-inflammatory properties make it good for delicate or scaly, damaged or itchy skin. It is also good in mouthwash for gingivitis. Myrrh can be used during childbirth to facilitate labour, and help prevent or treat postnatal infection of the reproductive system and it helps to tighten the tissues of the womb.
Contra-Indications	Safe to use in pregnancy and on children over two.
Main Therapeutic Properties	It is stimulant, anti-spasmodic, anaesthetic, anti-inflammatory and antiseptic. It stimulates the reproductive system, is anti-catarrhal, anti-fungal, anti-inflammatory, sedative and can treat gums and abscesses.
English Name	**MYRTLE**
Latin Name	*Myrtus communis*
Botanical Family	*Myrtaceae*
Description of Plant	Myrtle is an evergreen aromatic perennial shrub 1 to 3m high. It has shiny dark green leaves which are pointed and spiky with transparent glands. It produces odorous white solitary flowers.
Geographical Origin/Climate	Myrtle is commonly found in woods and scrubland in warm climates such as the Mediterranean area. It can be found growing right up to 800m of altitude in southern France. It is very common throughout Europe, in some parts of Asia and in North Africa.
Part Extracted for its Oil	Branches and leaves.
Method of Extraction	Distillation.
Chemical Constituents	Main chemical constituents: terpenoids: monoterpenes: camphene, cineole, geraniol, limonene, pinene, terpineol, myrtenol, nerol, linalol, terpinene; esters: terpinyl acetate,

continued overleaf

The Essential Oils *continued*

linalyl acetate, terpenyl, myrtenyl, neryl, geranyl, bornyl and carvyl acetate; sesquiterpenes: caryophyllene, caryophyllene oxide, humulene; aldehydes lactones: myrtucommulones.

Toxicity/Potential Hazards	None.
Key Qualities	Myrtle bestows divine grace.
Historical & Traditional Uses	Myrtle was a sacred tree to the Persians and is still revered in parts of Pakistan. Venus was said to be dressed with Myrtle leaves and the plant is one of her symbols.
Medicinal Activity	Myrtle is by far the best *Myrtaceae* for the treatment of asthma. It also helps pulmonary infections, bronchitis and sinusitis. Myrtle helps the circulation and is said to slow down internal bleeding. It is good for varicose veins and haemorrhoids. It is calming to the nervous system, much more gentle in its action than Eucalyptus, and therefore more suitable for children's ailments. It is a skin antiseptic, astringent and cicatrisant. Myrtle is recommended for urinary and genital infections. It is used to relieve rheumatic and arthritic pains.
Contra-Indications	Safe to use in therapeutic doses. Use on children over two.
Main Therapeutic Properties	Respiratory, nervous system, skin, digestion (gentle).
English Name	**NEROLI**
Latin Name	*Citrus auranthium* var. *amara*
Botanical Family	*Rutaceae*
Description of Plant	The bitter Seville Orange tree is an evergreen tree with shiny green leaves. It produces pure white odorant flowers that have five petals with many secretory oil sacs. The fruit is bright orange with a thick grainy rind and is the only tree to bear leaves, flowers and fruit at the same time.
Geographical Origin/Climate	Originally from China and India, Seville Orange is a small tree brought to Europe by the Crusaders. Many Mediterranean countries cultivate Orange trees and some are grown in orangeries as they don't like the cold winter. It is found in Israel, South Africa, Tunisia, France, Italy and Spain.
Part Extracted for its Oil	Flowers.
Method of Extraction	Distillation of freshly picked flowers.

Chemical Constituents	Main chemical constituents: terpenoids: monoterpenes: neryl acetate, geranyl acetate, linalyl acetate, pinene, limonene, linalol, geraniol, terpineol, nerol; sesquiterpenes: farnesol, nerolidol; aromatic alcohols: phenylethylic and benzylic alcohols; aldehydes: benzaldehyde; ketones: jasmone, indole.
Toxicity/Potential Hazards	None.
Key Qualities	Neroli is the scent that heals deep shock and trauma.
Historical & Traditional Uses	The word orange comes from the Arabic word *narandja*, itself stemming from the Sanskrit word *nagarunga*, meaning 'elephants' best fruit'. Under the name of Median apple, Theophrastus knew of an Orange tree originating from Asia and introduced by Alexander the Great. He described it as a tree with evergreen leaves, bearing inedible fruits, the skin of which was very perfumed. The famous 'golden apples' that Hippomen threw in the arena to run faster than the pretty Atalante were marvellous oranges stolen from the garden of the Hesperides. Neroli was named after Princess Nerola of Italy, who wore it as a perfume. Orange blossom is symbolic of chastity and virginity: the bride would traditionally wear an orange blossom headdress at her wedding; a dishonoured girl would not. In the south, conversely, Orange Flower water was the exclusive perfume of courtesans.
Medicinal Activity	Neroli anaesthetizes and is also a great hypnotizer. It is a stimulant of the parasympathetic nervous system and is very good for acute anxiety, upsets, fear, phobia, insomnia, psychotic states, panic attacks, epilepsy, hyperexcitability of reflexes and hyperactive states. Neroli calms and helps a person through difficult times. Cardiac problems: tachycardia pre and post cardiac surgery, high blood pressure. Calms down asthma, good for babies or very delicate skin, problems with digestion due to sensitivity and allergies (babies in particular).
Contra-Indications	Neroli: This oil is safe to use on everyone including babies. Be careful if using outdoor in the summer: it seems to attract bees, wasps and hornets, this is something that I have personally observed over many years.
Main Therapeutic Properties	Anti-depressant, antispasmodic, antiseptic, anxiolitic, anti-inflammatory, cicatrisant, hepatic, PMS, skin, digestive (babies), cardiac, blood pressure, deep stress, trauma.

The Essential Oils *continued*	
English Name	**NIAOULI**
Latin Name	*Melaleuca quinquinervia/veridiflora*
Botanical Family	*Myrtaceae*
Description of Plant	*Melaleuca quinquenervia* or *virdiflora* is a small evergreen tree and is a close relative of the Cajuput tree which it resembles and has many similar properties.
Geographical Origin/Climate	Niaouli is another subtropical tree which originates from New Caledonia and Austalia, but is now found in Madagascar, too.
Part Extracted for its Oil	Branches and leaves.
Method of Extraction	Distillation.
Chemical Constituents	Main chemical constituents: terpenoids: monoterpenes: linalol, terpineol, terpenene, cineole (38–58%), caryophellene; sesquiterpenes: globulol, viridiflorol, nerolidol, farnesols aldhydes: benzald and isovalerald.
Toxicity/Potential Hazards	Avoid use on babies and young children.
Key Qualities	Niaouli is the oil for serious ills.
Historical & Traditional Uses	Niaouli was imported to Europe in the 17th Century from New Caledonia under the name of Gomen oil, the name of the port of origin being Gomen.
Medicinal Activity	Niaouli has a stimulating effect when there is tissue damage; it stimulates local circulation, increases leucocytes and antibodies and stimulates tissue growth. It is very antiseptic and acts in a similar manner to some antibiotics and is a great help with infections. It has a beneficial effect on the respiratory system with bronchitis, flu, colds, rhinitis and TB. It also has a healing effect on the skin for conditions such as infected wounds or scars, ulcers, eczemas, psoriasis, shingles, furuncles, carbuncles, boils and abscesses. Finally, it is helpful for gynaecological problems and in pre- and post-surgery healing.
Contra-Indications	Should not be used in pregnancy, on young children and babies.
Main Therapeutic Properties	It is immuno-stimulant, anti-viral, anti-microbial, anti-bacterial, antibiotic, antiseptic, anti-infectious, anti-fungal, balsamic, cicatrisant and circulatory. It is also an emmenagogue and fights infections of the reproductive system.

English Name	**ORANGE (SWEET)**
Latin Name	*Citrus aurantium × sinensis*
Botanical Family	*Rutaceae*
Description of Plant	Evergreen shrub, which can grow up to 12m high. The small white fleshy flowers bloom during the whole year in warm countries. The orange fruit has an orange-yellow colour with lots of tiny essence vesicles just below the waxy surface. The taste of the orange is sweet.
Geographical Origin/Climate	Sweet Orange came from China, then to India, then Syria, Egypt and western Africa. It was brought to Europe at the time of the Crusades. It likes temperate to tropical climates. The Orange tree is cultivated in many areas with warm climates such as Israel, California, Florida, South Africa, Morocco, Spain and Greece.
Part Extracted for its Oil	Rind.
Method of Extraction	Expression.
Chemical Constituents	Main chemical constituents: coumarins and furanocoumarins: bergaptene, imperatorin, auraptene; monoterpenes: limonene 90 to 95%; linalol, myrcene, pinene; linalyl acetate; geraniol, terpineol; citral, citronellal; aliphatic aldehydes: C8, C10.
Toxicity/Potential Hazards	Photosensitive. Not to be applied to the skin prior to sunbathing. It may cause temporary pigmentation changes.
Key Qualities	Orange is a child's favourite.
Historical & Traditional Uses	Orange derives from the Arabic *narandja* and the Sanskrit *nagarunge* meaning 'elephants' best fruit'. *Sinensis* usually indicates that the plant originates from China. Greek mythology tells of the myth of the garden of the Hesperides where golden apples grew, possibly oranges or lemons. Orange is a symbol of sweetness. It used to be considered a handsome gift and was given at Christmas as a treat.
Medicinal Activity	It is of help to epilepsy sufferers, and also good for vertigo, palpitations, asthma and migraines. It facilitates digestion, particularly intestinal activity. It is good for IBS and constipation. It is a gentle sedative which works on anxiety, insomnia and severe nervousness. For the treatment of the skin, it is anti-wrinkle and good for oily skins, mouth ulcers and gingivitis.
Contra-Indications	Avoid sunbathing.

continued overleaf

The Essential Oils *continued*	
Main Therapeutic Properties	It is antiseptic, bactericide, carminative, astringent, purifying, regenerative, emollient, sedative and tonifying. It is also renowned for its skin softening virtues.

English Name	**PALMAROSA**
Latin Name	*Cymbopogon martinii*
Botanical Family	*Gramineae*
Description of Plant	It is a fragrant perennial grass which grows in tropical zones.
Geographical Origin/Climate	It grows in subtropical and tropical zones such as India, Africa, Java and Madagascar.
Part Extracted for its Oil	Aerial parts.
Method of Extraction	Distillation.
Chemical Constituents	Main chemical constituents: terpenoids: monoterpenes: limonene, phellandrene; geraniol (75 to 90%); esters: geranyl acetate and caproate, dipentene; carvone, citronellol, farnesol.
Toxicity/Potential Hazards	None known.
Key Qualities	Palmarosa brings softness and sensitivity.
Historical & Traditional Uses	For many years Palmarosa oil entered Europe via Turkey and was assumed to be Rose Geranium oil from Turkey. There two types of Palmarosa: *Motia* meaning precious and *Sophia* meaning mediocre, referring to the quality of the oil.
Medicinal Activity	It is a remedy for infectious illnesses involving fever. It is antiseptic and is excellent for skin care, and for dry and sensitive skin because of its hydrating properties. It helps acne, calms down itchy and burning sensations and encourages skin cell growth. It is indicated for mastitis, lymphatic congestion and water retention. Appropriate for pre- and post-labour pains and to help with general recovery as it is a tonic for the uterus. It is also good for the nervous system, and for postnatal depression and female hormone imbalances. It can help with panic attack palpitations. Can be used for emotional difficulties regarding fertility and conception as it is a very feminine oil.
Contra-Indications	Safe to use in therapeutic doses.
Main Therapeutic Properties	It is sedative, tonic, anti-depressant, neurotonic, hormone regulating, anti-fungal, antiseptic, anti-microbial, utero-tonic, lymphotonic, cicatrisant, healing, vulnerary, emollient, rehydrating.

English Name	**PATCHOULI**
Latin Name	*Pogostemon patchouli*
Botanical Family	*Labiatae/Lamiaceae*
Description of Plant	Patchouli is a herb which grows up to 1m in height with big oval leaves covered with hair from the secreting oil glands. It has white flowers; the plant has a strong but pleasant smell.
Geographical Origin/Climate	Cultivated in India, the Philippines, Java, Sumatra and Singapore.
Part Extracted for its Oil	Aerial parts.
Method of Extraction	Distillation.
Chemical Constituents	Main chemical constituents: terpenoids, monoterpenes; pinene, myrcene, sabinene, carene; sesquiterpenes: cadinenes, terpinene, cadinol; azulenes: patchoulene, norpatchoulenol.
Toxicity/Potential Hazards	None known.
Key Qualities	Patchouli awakens the longing for things from *le temps passé*.
Historical & Traditional Uses	When shawls were imported from India in the 1800s, their commercial success was such that the Scots decided to manufacture the same item from imported wools. These did not sell, and the merchants were both puzzled and disappointed. After enquiring with many ladies it was found that it was the scent in the shawls from India which made them more popular. After further enquiries, it was discovered that before departure from India the shawls were impregnated with Patchouli, to deter moths.
Medicinal Activity	The essential oil is fairly hypnotic and can induce a state of trance and it helps to bring about a meditative state. It contains may azulenes (patchoulene) which give it its special skin-healing properties. Good for acne, dermatitis, impetigo, shingles, herpes, allergies, ulcers, haemorrhoids.
Contra-Indications	Safe to use in therapeutic doses.
Main Therapeutic Properties	It is vulnerary and antiseptic (open wounds), anti-inflammatory, anti-pruritic, cicatrisant, healing, anti-fungal, bactericide; hypnotic, calming and protective (fortifying) and eases fluid retention.

The Essential Oils *continued*	
English Name	PEPPERMINT
Latin Name	*Mentha piperita*
Botanical Family	*Labiatae/Lamiaceae*
Description of Plant	Peppermint is a perennial plant which grows up to 70cm high and propagates itself by its roots and so tends to be fairly invasive. It produces small reddish or purple flowers. Peppermint is cultivated in France, Italy and Germany and in Michigan and Indiana in the United States. The best variety is often American Peppermint. There are two varieties of Peppermint: White and Black Peppermint.
Geographical Origin/Climate	Large quantities are grown in the USA. Also grown in China, Japan, India, Brazil, Russia and Spain.
Part Extracted for its Oil	Leaves.
Method of Extraction	Distillation.
Chemical Constituents	Main chemical constituents: lemonene (1 to 5%), menthol (30 to 55%), menthone (14 to 32%), 1,8-cineol, beta-phellandrine, menthofuran, limonene, menthylacetate (2 to 10%).
Toxicity/Potential Hazards	Can give palpitations and should be avoided with cardiac problems.
Key Qualities	Peppermint stimulates awareness and awakening.
Historical & Traditional Uses	Peppermint has been known as a medicinal plant since the days of Ancient Egypt for the fresh sensation it creates. Hippocrates mentions its use as a stimulant for the treatment of acute illnesses. Pliny commented that Peppermint has a smell which wakes you up and excites the appetite. Widely cultivated for its fine essence, Peppermint has an aromatic and pervasive scent. Its taste, hot and peppery at first, leaves a pleasant, refreshing sensation. All Peppermints cultivated in England and elsewhere are said to have come from a unique plant, in Mitcham, Surrey. Although the plantation does not exist any more, Mitcham Peppermint represents quality Peppermint.
Medicinal Activity	The leaves and the oil from the Peppermint plant are used to ease painful periods and abdominal cramps. It is an emmenagogue and the tea is taken to bring on periods. Peppermint when applied locally can soothe and relieve itchy sensations caused by skin infections or inflammation.

	It is a first-aid oil for treating insect stings and bites, particularly bees and wasps. It is a deodorant and is useful for mouth hygiene, gingivitis and sore throats. It is a powerful astringent and tightens up the skin. It is also antiseptic and anti-bacterial. It is a cardiac stimulant and can make the heart beat faster in people in a state of anxiety. It eases digestion and recovery from food poisoning. It helps intestinal pains caused by diarrhoea and stimulates urination. It is used extensively for colds and flu, helps spasmodic coughs, relieves blocked nose symptoms and sinusitis.
Contra-Indications	Not to used in pregnancy, should be well diluted for children, not to be used with children under five.
Main Therapeutic Properties	Peppermint clears the mind and helps concentrate when 100% attention is needed. Peppermint has diuretic, choleretic, carminative, digestive and aperitive properties. It is renowned for its anti-tussive, sudorific, expectorant and decongestant properties. It is a vasoconstrictor, anti-coagulant, cardiac stimulant and is good for varicose veins. For the skin it is anti-inflammatory, analgesic and anti-pruritic, anti-bacterial, anti-viral, anti-fungal, antiseptic, deodorant, refreshing and a general tonic.
English Name	**PETITGRAIN**
Latin Name	*Citrus aurantium* var. *amara*
Botanical Family	*Rutaceae*
Description of Plant	The *Citrus aurantium* is another evergreen tree of the citrus family which grows in warm regions.
Geographical Origin/Climate	Petitgrain grows in Mediterranean countries, Paraguay, Africa and Israel.
Part Extracted for its Oil	Stems and leaves.
Method of Extraction	Distillation.
Chemical Constituents	Main chemical constituents: terpenoids: monoterpenes: myrcene, cymene, ocimene; esters: (50 to 80%) – linolyl acetate; neryl acetate, terpenyl acetate, geranyl acetate; alcohols: geraniol, linalol, terpineol, nerol.
Toxicity/Potential Hazards	None in therapeutic doses. Not for sunbathing.
Key Qualities	Petitgrain is the remedy to cure thoughts that go around in the mind.

continued overleaf

The Essential Oils *continued*	
Historical & Traditional Uses	*See* Neroli.
Medicinal Activity	Petitgrain is a gentle sedative and works on the nervous system, a bit like Neroli, to which it is related, and Mandarin. It is good for shocks, trauma, stress, exhaustion and depression. It also works on neuralgia, nervous pains, cramps, digestive spasms, insomnia and nightmares.
Contra-Indications	Non-toxic and safe to use on everyone.
Main Therapeutic Properties	It is relaxing, tonic, sedative, hypnotic, anti-epileptic, anti-spasmodic, anti-inflammatory and antiseptic.
English Name	PINE
Latin Name	*Pinus sylvestris*
Botanical Family	*Conifera/Pinaceae*
Description of Plant	The Pine tree is a pyramid-shaped, majestic tree which can grow to 30m high. It has sharp and prickly needles.
Geographical Origin/Climate	Pine trees are still very common in the wild as well as being widely cultivated. It tends to grow in any climate, whether high mountains or cold plains, and it can withstand temperatures as low as –40°C. There are Siberian and Finnish Pines, but the ones used for oil are Siberian.
Part Extracted for its Oil	Fresh needles.
Method of Extraction	Distillation.
Chemical Constituents	Main chemical constituents: esters: bornyl acetate (30 to 40%), monoterpenes: cadinene, lemonenes, pinenes, sylvestrene and borneol; sesquiterpenes: cadinol.
Toxicity/Potential Hazards	None.
Key Qualities	Pine is the oil that speaks of adventures.
Historical & Traditional Uses	Hippocrates recommended it against illnesses of the lungs, and Avicenna, a famous Arab physician, talked about its merits at length in one of his medical treatises. Pliny recommended it as a pectoral and expectorant and talked about the different species of Pine.
Medicinal Activity	Pine oil tends to stimulate the metabolism. It increases excretion, stamina release and cardiovascular activity. It also encourages blood circulation and tends to be hypertensive. Its diuretic activity helps prevent formation of kidney stones. It helps cystitis, thrush, bladder and kidney

	infections. As an antiseptic and expectorant, it helps clear mucous and fight colds and flu, treats pneumonia, bronchitis and asthma and heals lung tissues. It stimulates secretion of adrenocorticosteroid hormones. It can be used on children over five as its action is fairly gentle. Pine is fast-acting and has a characteristically light, short-lived activity and is excreted quickly.
Contra-Indications	It is a safe oil to use in therapeutic doses. It can be used for children over five and is safe in pregnancy unless there is high blood pressure.
Main Therapeutic Properties	It is antiseptic, anti-viral, antibiotic, anti-fungal, diuretic and sudorific. It is also a surrenal hormone stimulant, a neurotonic, general tonic, lympho-tonic and tonic for the urinary and reproductive system. It is hypertensive, anti-diabetes, expectorant and pectoral.

English Name	**ROSE**	**ROSE (Absolute)**
Latin Name	*Rosa damascena* (Otte or Attar of Roses)	*Rosa centifolia*
Botanical Family	*Rosaceae*	
Description of Plant	There are hundreds of roses growing all over the northern hemisphere and they all evolved from a few very ancient roses. Rose Damask is of Syrian origin while the *centifolia* is a descendant of the Persian rose, the famous rose of Ispahan. Roses are either climbers or standing bushes with indented green leaves that in some instances can also be distilled for their oil. The petals are large in size and the smell very odorant.	
Geographical Origin/Climate	Roses grow all over the northern hemisphere, but the ones for the oil are cultivated in Turkey, Bulgaria and Morocco.	
Part Extracted for its Oil	Petals.	Petals/rose leaves.
Method of Extraction	Distillation.	Solvent extraction.
Chemical Constituents	Main chemical constituents (rose distillation): phenols: eugenol; terpenoids: monoterpenes: myrcene, pinene; alcohols (50%): citronellol, nerol, geraniol, linalol; geranyl acetate; citral; carvone and sesquiterpenes: farnesol and natural waxes.	
Toxicity/Potential Hazards	None, Rose is the least toxic of all oils.	Can be a mild skin irritant.

continued overleaf

133

The Essential Oils *continued*		
Key Qualities	Rose carries the soul back to the garden.	
Historical & Traditional Uses	The word *rosae* is said to a Latin adaptation of the celtic word *rhod*, meaning red. *Centifolia* means hundreds of leaves or petals. Rosaries are strings of beads representing the many spiritual prayer offerings to the Virgin Mary. Troubadours associated the rose with perfect beauty and purity of heart as in true love. Jehangir Khan, a Mogul Emperor from Persian India, had thousands of rose petals scattered over the moat of his fortress on his wedding day. By the end of the day it was noticed that the water looked illuminated by the setting sun to the great amazement of the guests. It was discovered later on that this phenomenon was due to the wax and the oil distilled from the rose petals which reflected the sunlight as if it was a powerful mirror. Nicholas Culpeper refers to it in his herbal as a remedy for the convected heart. People used to make rose-petal jam to use as a laxative.	
Medicinal Activity	Rose is the 'Queen of the garden' and the 'Essence of love', but also the oil for sorrow. Rose can reach the very essence of our being and mellow inner turmoil. It is a tonic for the heart and is highly recommended for emotional or physical heart problems. Rose works on the circulation and helps treat broken surface capillaries. It is a gentle antiseptic for the chest and is indicated when a person is in a delicate state of health. It helps severe asthma sufferers, bronchitis and pneumonia. It soothes the lungs and respiratory membranes. It is very healing for all types of skin but more particularly for damaged, mature or allergic skins. It is also good for skin ulcers.	
Contra-Indications	Rose distillation: one of the least toxic oils, it is very safe to use on everyone.	Rose Absolute: all absolutes should only be used for their wondrous scent as usually the extraction procedure for absolutes does not distort the odour in the way the distillation process does. Therapeutically, it benefits the mind by the interaction of the essential oil's odour with the sense of smell. One to two drops are usually enough in a blend. Other absolute essential oils are: Jasmine, Violet, Gardenia, Mimosa, Carnation.

Main Therapeutic Properties	Cardiac, nervous system, psychic unbalance, grief, obsessions, gynaecological disorders, deep stress and anxiety, shocks, not hepato-toxic. It is cicatrisant, astringent, emollient, moisturizing.
English Name	**ROSEMARY**
Latin Name	*Rosmarinus officinalis*
Botanical Family	*Labiatae/Lamiaceae*
Description of Plant	Rosemary is a perennial evergreen plant; it produces little white, pink or sky-blue flowers depending on the species and type of soil it grows in. It grows into a handsome shrub which can reach up to 2m high.
Geographical Origin/Climate	Rosemary flowers most of the year when growing in warm climates. It grows wild at low altitude in dry and arid areas: scrublands and stony grounds mostly near the sea coast of the Mediterranean. It is also widely cultivated in countries like Spain, North Africa, and so on.
Part Extracted for its Oil	Flowering tops, leaves.
Method of Extraction	Distillation. Often adulterated with Spanish Eucalyptus oil.
Chemical Constituents	Main chemical constituents: terpenoids: monoterpenes (25–40%); limonene, camphene, terpinene, pinene, phellandrene, cymene; isobornyl acetate; alcohols: borneol, 15% camphor, 15 to 30% cineole, geraniol, linalol, terpineol, verbenol, safrol, verbenone.
Toxicity/Potential Hazards	Should be used only in therapeutic doses and not over prolonged periods of time.
Key Qualities	Rosemary is the great energizer.
Historical & Traditional Uses	Rosemary comes from *rosemarinus*, from the Latin *ros*, meaning, dew, and *marinus* from *mare*, meaning sea; 'rose from the sea' refers to the fact that it grows on the sea coast. Rosemary has been renowned for its culinary, medicinal and magical properties and has been used often for religious ceremonies and festivals. Considered sacred in many civilizations, Rosemary is one of the oldest plants used in herbal pharmacopoeia, and was employed in abundance during times of plague and epidemics to drive away evil spirits. 'Rosemary for remembrance' is a saying with regard to the herb, which was once popular in times of mourning. It was also associated with rebirth and was used in the bridal bouquet.

continued overleaf

The Essential Oils *continued*	
Medicinal Activity	Rosemary stimulates the senses, its action being most beneficial for physical invigoration, 'bringing you to your senses'. It increases stamina and can help chronic fatigue syndrome or just lack of energy after illness. It is one of the best oils for convalescence. It is also good for the despondency type of depression. It helps when people feel they lack the courage to do something. It is very good for sprains, muscle injuries, cramps, myalgia and recovery from bone fractures. It is good for low blood pressure and has a very cleansing effect on the digestive system. It is sudorific, diuretic, mucolytic and is indispensable if trying to lose weight. It is a decongestant of the lymphatic and venous system. It is a fast-acting oil and should be used in moderation. It is used as a hair conditioner as well as in face masks for acne.
Contra-Indications	Inhaling too much can cause nausea and disorientation. Strongly stimulates the nervous system. Not to be used in pregnancy and children under ten and not on babies. Not for people with high blood pressure.
Main Therapeutic Properties	It is a nervous stimulant and a good tonic and it is an antidepressant. It has good expectorant properties, is cardiotonic, hypertensive; a muscular anti-spasmodic and relaxant, is sudorific, diuretic, anti-arthritic and anti-rheumatic. It is prophylactic, digestive, hepatic, choleretic, cholegogue and a hair tonic.
English Name	**ROSEWOOD**
Latin Name	*Aniba rosaedora*
Botanical Family	*Lauracea*
Description of Plant	Rosewood is an evergreen medium-sized tree, its wood is a reddish colour and produces leathery green leaves and small yellow flowers.
Geographical Origin/Climate	Rosewood is native to subtropical Amazonia. It mainly grows in Brazil, Peru and Guyana.
Part Extracted for its Oil	Chipped wood.
Method of Extraction	Distillation.
Chemical Constituents	Main chemical constituents: terpenoids: monoterpenes: 10% cineole, citronellal, geraniol, limonene, linalol (60 to 90%), pinene, terpineol and elemene.
Toxicity/Potential Hazards	None known.

Key Qualities	Rosewood induces a cheerful mood.
Historical & Traditional Uses	Rosewood's species name, *rosaedora*, probably relates to its subtle scent of rose.
Medicinal Activity	Rosewood is one of the most uplifting and cheering of oils. It is indicated where there is physical and emotional trauma like physical abuse, assault etc., or when there is fear of intimacy and sexual disability. Rosewood is very antiseptic and particularly good for ear, nose and throat infections. It is recommended for inflammation of the lymph vessels (lymphangitis).
Contra-Indications	None when used in therapeutic dosage.
Main Therapeutic Properties	It is an anti-viral, anti-bacterial and anti-fungal agent. It has anti-spasmodic, deodorant, anti-allergic, anti-aging, antiseptic properties and helps with gynaecological and sexual problems. It is also a tonic, an anti-depressant and a mood enhancer.
English Name	**SANDALWOOD**
Latin Name	*Santalum album*
Botanical Family	*Santalaceae*
Description of Plant	The *Santalum album* is an evergreen tree indigenous to the hills of Mysore which can grow from 8 to 10m high. The tree is parasitic as it attaches its roots to the nearby vegetation and draws its nourishment from it, eventually causing the death of the host plants. When cultivated it needs to be planted with other trees in order to survive. Only the heartwood of fully mature and naturally dying trees are used for distillation.
Geographical Origin/Climate	*Santalum album* is essentially an equatorial plant as the closer to the equator the finer its essential oil. It likes the habitat of stony ground in arid mountainous areas. It is cultivated in India, New Caledonia and Indonesia. Genuine Mysore Sandalwood is getting rarer as it is only available from the region of Karnataka and Tamil Nadu, south-east India and there is great demand for it from all over the world.
Part Extracted for its Oil	Heartwood taken from an 18- to 25-year old tree.
Method of Extraction	Steam distillation.
Chemical Constituents	Main chemical constituents: terpenoids: monoterpenes: borneol, sesquiterpene alcohols: 90 to 97% santalols, santalyl acetate; sesquiterpenes: santalenes, curcumenes, farnesene, santol, santolone, santanol.

continued overleaf

The Essential Oils *continued*	
Toxicity/Potential Hazards	None when used in therapeutic doses.
Key Qualities	Sandalwood protects the purity of the soul.
Historical & Traditional Uses	Sandal derives from the Latin *santalum*, an adaptation of the Indian word *santal*. In India the *santal* tree is referred to as *cadana* (from the Sanskrit), meaning generous. Its wondrous smell makes it important in spiritual practices in India and all over the Asian world as it is burned in most temples. The Sandal tree is one of the Heavenly trees and many sacred objects are made of Sandalwood in India and Tibet as it represents the radiance of the Gods.
Medicinal Activity	It is mildly sedative and hypnotic and calms excessive behaviour, particularly excessive pride. In South India its powder is mixed with Tumeric to keep the brain cool while working in the heat in the field. It is very good for delirium, nightmares and something the Victorians called 'brain fever' (temporary madness). Recent research has shown the possibility that the oil is chemoprotective in cases of liver cancer and it is still being investigated. Particularly good as a decongestant for the circulatory system.
Contra-Indications	It is safe to use on everyone in therapeutic doses.
Main Therapeutic Properties	It is sedative, calming, analgesic, anti-infectious, diuretic, emollient, cicatrisant, astringent, soothing to the skin, anti-inflammatory and tonic.
English Name	TEA TREE
Latin Name	*Melaleuca alternifolia*
Botanical Family	*Myrtaceae*
Description of Plant	It is an evergreen which can reach 8m in height. It has narrow, soft, needle-shaped leaves. The leaves have a similar smell to Eucalyptus, but more subtle.
Geographical Origin/Climate	Tea Tree is part of the *Melaleuca* family and a cousin of Eucalyptus. It grows in tropical areas. It is native of the subtropical area in Bangawalbyn, New South Wales and Queensland in Australia. Also found in South Africa, India and Malaysia. There are around 300 different species of Tea Tree. Other Tea Tree species which have raised a lot of interest in recent times are Red and White Manuka.
Part Extracted for its Oil	Leaves and twigs.

Method of Extraction	Steam distillation.
Chemical Constituents	Main chemical constituents: terpenoids: monoterpenes: cymene, limonene, pinene, terpinene, terpinolene: alcohols: 3.5% to 8% cineole, terpineol 30 to 40%, thyunol, viridiflorol; sesquiterpenes: viridiflorene, cadinene, aromadendrene. Note that Tea Tree oil is widely adulterated or synthetized.
Toxicity/Potential Hazards	Non-toxic.
Key Qualities	Tea Tree is medication for mental and physical illnesses due to external causes.
Historical & Traditional Uses	Aborigines in Australia have made use of Tea Tree for thousands of years. They use the crushed leaves on all sorts of infected wounds. It was early settlers in Australia who extracted its essential oil and it was widely used by the Australian Army as a 'cure for all' when camping out in the bush. Some of the problems Tea Tree is known to be excellent for are: insect bites and poison, leech bites, sunburn, infected small wounds, skin parasites. Tea Tree owes its name to Captain Cook's crew, who ran out of tea while in Australia and began to use Tea Tree leaves instead. It was in the 1920s that the amazing antiseptic properties of Tea Tree were brought to light, but it was not until 1976 that an Australian family decided to cultivate the Tea Tree.
Medicinal Activity	There are two definite chemotypes of Tea Tree: one smells a little bit like nutmeg because of its higher terpineol (40%) content and has a superior overall healing power and can boost the immune system. The other chemotype smells strongly of camphor because of its high cineole (8%) content and tends to be better at fighting colds and flu. The cineole chemotype is known to be a powerful mucous membrane and skin irritant. The cineole chemotype should not be more than 8% in its composition to avoid irritation. Their properties overlap, however, and for the treatment of many small ills as long as it is a genuine Tea Tree oil it will work out positively. Minor sexually transmitted diseases can also be treated with Tea Tree alongside pharmaceutical medication. Gynaecological infections like thrush, pelvic inflammation, and post-labour tears can be treated with Tea Tree.
Contra-Indications	Non-toxic and can be used on everyone in therapeutic doses.

continued overleaf

The Essential Oils *continued*

Main Therapeutic Properties	Highly antiseptic, anti-fungal, anti-viral, anti-bacterial, anti-infectious, anti-inflammatory, cicatrisant, vulnerary and healing properties. It has immuno-stimulant and anti-parasitic properties. It also has decongestant, pectoral, depurative, expectorant, sudorific and diuretic properties.
English Name	**THYME**
Latin Name	*Thymus vulgaris*
Botanical Family	*Labiatae/Lamiaceae*
Description of Plant	Thyme is a fairly small shrub which grows wild in the south of France and many other Mediterranean countries. It produces tiny white or pink flowers.
Geographical Origin/Climate	Thyme grows in dry and arid places in many temperate and subtropical zones. It is cultivated in France, Spain, Portugal, Greece and in California, USA.
Part Extracted for its Oil	Flowering stems and tops.
Method of Extraction	Distillation.
Chemical Constituents	Main chemical constituents: phenols: 30 to 40% thymol, 2.5 to 15% carvacrol, cymol; terpenoids: monoterpenes: camphene, limonene, linalol, pinene, terpinene; alcohols: borneol, terpineol, geraniol, linalol, cineole and esters: geranyl acetate; sesquiterpenes: caryophyllene.
Toxicity/Potential Hazards	In high doses or repeated uses can be neurotoxic, strongly emmenagogue and hypertensor.
Key Qualities	Thyme curbs excesses.
Historical & Traditional Uses	*Thymus* is an old Greek name used by Theophrastus to refer to Thyme or Savoury. Another name for this plant was the 'shepherdess grass' as it was believed to protect chastity. The Egyptians used it with other aromatic plants for embalming. Theophrastus, Dioscorides and Gallen all talk of its virtues and its digestive and anti-infectious properties.
Medicinal Activity	Thyme is a constitutional remedy which works on many deep processes. It can help strengthen weak organs after illness or fight illnesses caused by infection. It is a nervous tonic and stimulant and is recommended for people with compulsive personalities or disorders. Its ability to clear physical congestion can also be translated as clearing psychological congestion as it makes people more 'open'. Wild Thyme is often an ingredient in ointment for sport

	injuries and it has an anti-inflammatory capacity when used on rheumatism and sprains. It helps to clear the 'backlog' of waste products and encourages fluid reabsorption. It is excellent for losing weight and detoxifying. It stimulates capillarial circulation and brings on periods. It is good for the skin, particularly for sebaceous conditions like acne or boils. It has astringent, antiseptic, anti-fungal properties. It is a skin disinfectant and clears bacterial and parasitic infections.
Contra-Indications	Not to be used in pregnancy, for children and babies, and not when there is high blood pressure.
Main Therapeutic Properties	Thyme is renowned for its carminative, digestive, anti-spasmodic and cholagogue properties. It is a powerful sudorific, emmenagogue and diuretic. It is highly anti-infectious, anti-bacterial, anti-viral, an expectorant and anti-inflammatory. It is a strong hypertensor.
English Names	(LEMON) VERBENA
Latin Name	*Lippia citriodora*
Botanical Family	*Verbenaceae*
Description of Plant	This small tree can grow up to 8m, although is usually slightly smaller in cooler temperate zones. The smell of the leaves is delicate and hypnotic; it produces tiny, exquisite flowers which are bluish-white and packed in spiky clusters.
Geographical Origin/Climate	Native to Chile and Peru, Lemon Verbena does not withstand frost. It has been introduced into Spain, northern Africa, India, Réunion Island and Australia where it is commonly cultivated.
Part Extracted for its Oil	Branches and leaves.
Method of Extraction	Distillation.
Chemical Constituents	Main chemical constituents: monoterpenes: 30 to 35% citral, limonene, linalol, geraniol, nerol, terpineol and cineole; sesquiterpenes: caryophyllene.
Toxicity/Potential Hazards	None known.
Key Qualities	Verbena is the oil that restores clarity.
Historical & Traditional Uses	Verbena is said to have been given its Latin name, *lippia*, after a prominent 17th-century botanist. It is said that a bath with Verbena leaves purifies body and soul. It was one of the ingredients in magic love potions.

continued overleaf

The Essential Oils *continued*	
Medicinal Activity	Verbena gives clarity and lucidity and helps decrease 'hyper' symptoms; it is a tonic for the nervous system. Verbena is indicated for states of hysteria, it is also good for insomnia, depression and nervous exhaustion. Verbena is a favourite scent with men and is included in countless aftershave recipes. It is recommended for tachycardia, coronary disease and hypertension. Lemon Verbena helps digestive problems caused by nervousness or anxiety. Finally, it can be used for diabetics, Crohn's disease and Hodgkin's disease.
Contra-Indications	Can cause skin irritation on people with a pronounced skin allergy. Not to be used on children under ten and babies.
Main Therapeutic Properties	It has tonic, anti-inflammatory, anti-spasmodic, sedative, analgesic and neuro-muscular properties. It is also a digestive, eupeptic and carminative, and stimulates hepatic, spleenic and pancreatic functions. It is a stimulant to both ovaries and testes. It regulates thyroid activity. It has purifying, tonifying and refreshing properties. It is a hypotensor.
English Name	VETIVERT/Vetyvert
Latin Name	*Vetiveria zizanoides*
Botanical Family	*Gramineae*
Description of Plant	The plant is a tall, perennial grass with strong roots by which it propagates itself.
Geographical Origin/Climate	It likes to grow in volcanic sands and ashes. In fact, in parts of India which are prone to spontaneous fires it is used as a fire-break. This is because the top part of the plant will burn but the deep, tough roots will resist and so slow down the spread of the fire.
Part Extracted for its Oil	Root.
Method of Extraction	Distillation.
Chemical Constituents	Main chemical constituents: vetivenol (60%), vetivenone (13%), vetivene, retivenylacetate, vetivazulene.
Toxicity/Potential Hazards	None known.
Key Qualities	Vetivert brings peace and stability.
Historical & Traditional Uses	Vetivert when fresh has an earthy scent of freshly dug-up

	potatoes. In India the roots of Vetivert are woven into fine mats and sprayed with water to reproduce the scent of the damp earth after the rain, creating a sensation of coolness. In Réunion people make large fans which exude their scent every time the wind blows through them.
Medicinal Activity	It is recommended for anxiety and insomnia, regulates some of the deep processes of the autonomic nervous system, can be helpful with psychosomatic ailments, psychiatric conditions, agitation and delusion. It is used for skin care, for sores, insect bites and as an insect repellent.
Contra-Indications	Non-toxic, but it has a very penetrating pungent smell and should be used sparingly in a blend as it tends to overpower the other smells.
Main Therapeutic Properties	It has sedative, sudorific, diaphoretic, cicatrisant and healing properties.
English Name	**VIOLET**
Latin Name	*Viola odorata*
Botanical Family	*Violaceae*
Description of Plant	The plant grows to about 10 to 30cm high, is herbaceous and perennial. Violets have small flowers with five petals, all of different sizes. They can be light or dark purple and have heart-shaped leaves. The plants tend to blossom from February to May but need a good frost in the winter to flower properly. The flowers give a very delicate fragrance and the leaves are also scented but to a lesser degree.
Geographical Origin/Climate	One of 'heralds' of spring, Violets grow naturally in pastures, woods and hedges. Violet is native to Britain and is cultivated in Europe, western Asia, India and northern Africa.
Part Extracted for its Oil	Flowers/leaves.
Method of Extraction	Solvent extraction. 'Absolute'.
Chemical Constituents	Main chemical constituents: phenols: eugenol; ketones: parmone, ionone, methyl ionone, irone; hexenic, octonic and benzylic alcohol, esanol.
Toxicity/Potential Hazards	None known.
Key Qualities	Violet is the symbol of subtle beauty.

continued overleaf

The Essential Oils *continued*

Historical & Traditional Uses	The name Viola derives from the Greek *io* meaning violet. The Greeks believed that if they wore Violet wreaths on their head they could drink as much as they wanted and not get drunk. Theophrastus refers to it in his work. Mohamed, the prophet, compares the superior qualities of God to the superior perfume of the Violet over other flowers.
Medicinal Activity	Violet is effective against coughs, itching sensations due to skin infections (scratches, breaks, cracks) and against insect stings and bites. It has softening, moisturizing and purifying properties. The essential oil is renowned for its antiseptic virtues. It is good for sensitive and irritated skin suffering from acne and for after-sun products.
Contra-Indications	No known contra-indications.
Main Therapeutic Properties	It has analgesic, sedative and anti-inflammatory properties. It is also used for its anti-tussive, expectorant and decongestant properties for the respiratory tracts.
English Name	**YLANG-YLANG**
Latin Name	*Cananga odorata*
Botanical Family	*Annonaceae*
Description of Plant	When adult, the tree can reach 20m high and has a very erect stem, with more or less horizontal branches, the lower ones dangling. It is an evergreen tree. The flowers make clusters all through the year so they can always be harvested, but the nicest are in bloom during winter. Whitish-green at first, they then turn yellow. The fruit is a fleshy oblong pod, green when young, black when mature. The flowers are used. They must be harvested when yellow and emit a strong, pleasant smell. An essential oil is extracted from them after steam distillation.
Geographical Origin/Climate	Ylang-Ylang is a weeping tree native to the Philippines. Fond of damp, warm climates but unable to stand violent winds, Ylang-Ylang is nowadays cultivated in Indonesia and on the Comoro Islands. It was introduced in the Réunion in 1884. The Japanese destroyed the Ylang-Ylang on the Philippines during the Second World War.
Part Extracted for its Oil	Flowers.
Method of Extraction	Distillation.

Chemical Constituents	Main chemical constituents: phenols: eugenol; terpenoids: monoterpenes: pinene, geraniol, linalol; sesquiterpenes: caryophyllene, cadinene, farnesol; esters: geronyl and boznylacetate.
Toxicity/Potential Hazards	The smell is very strong and the oil should be used sparingly.
Key Qualities	Ylang-Ylang seduces the heart into intimacy.
Historical & Traditional Uses	*Cananga* is derived from the word *kanonga*, the name given to Ylang-Ylang by natives of Borneo; it means 'flower of the flowers'. In the Far East, Ylang-Ylang was traditionally used to protect against the cold and rainy season. The flowers were added to cocoa butter and made into an ointment that people rubbed on their body to keep them healthy.
Medicinal Activity	Ylang-Ylang works its magic on the chest where it calms downs the breathing rhythm, and is especially effective for bad coughs. It has been found to regulate parasympathetic activity and is recommended for nervous problems such as nervous tension, high anxiety, grief, shock and trauma, hypersensitivity and hyperexcitability and epilepsy. It also helps regulate cardiac rhythm and lowers high blood pressure. It increases sensuality and is useful in treating frigidity or impotence. It is a skin antiseptic, good for oily skin and acne; it is also good for sensitive and delicate skin, and promotes hair growth.
Contra-Indications	Inhaling strong doses can cause nausea, headaches, trembling and deplete the nervous system, making you feel tired.
Main Therapeutic Properties	Ylang-Ylang has sedative, hypotensive, calmative and anti-spasmodic properties. It is also antiseptic, anti-fungal and anti-bacterial.

Ailments of the Cardiac System

List of Ailments	Definition	Therapeutic Guide	Choice of Essential Oils	Contra-Indications and Cautions	Treatment
Angina Pectoris	Failure of the coronary arteries to provide sufficient. oxygen to the heart muscle. Tightness and acute pain from the centre of the chest radiating to the neck and down the left arm. Caused by arteriosclerosis, this serious condition denotes diseased coronary arteries and needs to be medically monitored. Other symptoms will be: diminished cardiac activity and high blood pressure. Emotional factors can also contribute to the acuteness of the condition.	Vasodilator, anti-coagulant, anti-spasmodic.	**Angelica,** Lavender, **Lemon,** Neroli, Rose, Ylang-Ylang.	Angelica increases photosensitivity and should not be used in pregnancy.	**Gentle aromatic massage.**
Hypertension	Abnormally raised blood pressure. Can be caused by other diseases such as diabetes or by deterioration of parts of the cardio-vascular system. Can also be stress-related and is more likely to occur in the older person.	Hypotensives, myorelaxants, diuretics, anti-stress.	Angelica, **Geranium,** Lemon, Lavender, Rose, **Marjoram,** Ylang-Ylang.	Angelica and Lemon increase photosensitivity and Angelica should not be used during pregnancy.	**Gentle aromatic massage.**

List of Ailments	Definition	Therapeutic Guide	Choice of Essential Oils	Contra-Indications and Cautions	Treatment
Hypotension	An abnormally low blood pressure due to illness or extreme weakness.	Hypertensors, rubefacient, warming.	**Black Pepper, Cinnamon, Ginger,** Juniper, Pine, **Rosemary, Thyme.**	These oils should not be used during pregnancy.	**Swedish massage** with essential oils to energize the body.
Palpitations (Tachycardia)	An abnormal, rapid or irregular heartbeat. Can be caused by a cardiac defect but in many instances is stress-related.	Anti-stress, anxiolytic, myorelaxant, nerve relaxant.	Lavender, Lemon, **Marjoram, Melissa, Neroli,** Petitgrain, **Rose,** Ylang-Ylang.	Lemon increases photosensitivity.	**Aromatic massage bath** and **vaporization.**

Ailments of the Circulatory System

List of Ailments	Definition	Therapeutic Guide	Choice of Essential Oils	Contra-Indications and Cautions	Treatment
Chilblains	Hot, red, swollen and very itchy patches of skin on the hands, fingers, toes and ears caused by repeated exposure to heat or cold.	Vasoconstrictor, anti-inflammatory, decongestant.	Cypress, Geranium, **Juniper,** Mandarin, Palmarosa, Patchouli.	Cypress and Juniper should not be used in pregnancy or where there is a high blood pressure condition.	Virgin olive oil with essential oils need to be massaged onto the affected areas.
Fluid Congestion in Legs	Fluid retention in the legs will cause the legs to swell and may be caused by varicose veins or phlebitis.	Lymphatic decongestant, anti-oedematous, diuretics, sudorifics.	Cedarwood, Cypress, **Clary Sage, Fennel,** Geranium, Grapefruit, **Juniper,** Lemon, Palmarosa.	Cedarwood, Cypress, Clary Sage, Fennel and Juniper should not be used during pregnancy. Cypress, Clary Sage, Fennel and Juniper should not be used where there is high blood pressure.	**Lymphatic massage** of the legs. **Aromatic baths** if caused by varicose veins or phlebitis.

147

Ailments of the Circulatory System *continued*

List of Ailments	Definition	Therapeutic Guide	Choice of Essential Oils	Contra-Indications and Cautions	Treatment
Phlebitis	Inflammation of a vein causing the leg to swell drastically. It is very painful. It may cause the formation of a blood clot, a serious condition called thrombophlebitis.	Anti-inflammatories, phlebo-tonic, anti-coagulants, tonic of the lymphatic system.	Angelica, Cedarwood, **Cinnamon**, Geranium, Myrtle, Neroli, Niaouli, Lavender, Lime, Tea Tree.	Angelica and Lime increase photosensitivity. Angelica and Cinnamon should not be used during pregnancy.	Blend an aqueous base lotion with the essential oils and apply lightly and regularly. **No massage.**
Varicose Veins	Defective vascular mechanism causes congestion in the veins of the legs, eventually damaging the vein structure and causing swelling of veins. It can be caused by pregnancy, obesity, occupations requiring standing up for long periods, excessive exertion of the legs and poor circulation.	Anti-inflammatory, vasoconstrictors.	**Camomile**, Cypress, **Geranium, Juniper.**	Cypress and Juniper should not be used in pregnancy or where there is high blood pressure.	Blend an aqueous cream lotion with the oils and apply regularly or use the essential oils blended in virgin olive oil and apply to the leg but do not massage.

Ailments of the Digestive System

List of Ailments	Definition	Therapeutic Guide	Choice of Essential Oils	Contra-Indications and Cautions	Treatment
Burning Acidity (Heartburn)	An unusually high level of gastric juices (acid) in the upper part of the stomach which causes a sense of	Stomachic, digestive, calmative.	Angelica, **Aniseed**, Bergamot, Coriander, **Lemon Grass**, Lemon	Angelica, Aniseed and Peppermint should not be used during pregnancy and	Localized aromatic massage in the epigastric region of the abdomen.

THERAPEUTIC GUIDE TO ESSENTIAL OILS

Condition	Description	Properties	Oils	Precautions	Application
	...burning and discomfort.		Verbena and Peppermint.	Angelica, Aniseed, Bergamot and Lemon all increase photosensitivity.	Localized aromatic massage in the affected area of the abdomen.
Colitis	Inflammation and ulceration of the small or large intestine It is often a stress-related disorder.	Antiseptic, spasmolytic, anti-bacterial, anti-inflammatory, myorelaxant, anti-stress.	Aniseed, Basil, Camomile, Clary Sage, Marjoram, Lemon Grass, Lemon Verbena, Peppermint, Thyme.	Aniseed, Basil, Clary Sage, Peppermint and Thyme should not be used during pregnancy. Basil, Peppermint and Thyme should not be used where there is high blood pressure.	Localized aromatic massage in the affected area of the lower abdomen. After each meal, it is recommended to drink the corresponding herbal tea to the oils used, if available.
Dyspepsia (Indigestion)	Any disruptive symptoms that cause painful digestion, spasms, sensations of 'bloatedness' or fullness or general discomfort. This is not connected to heart problems. This problem can be stress-related.	Stomachic, spasmolytic, digestive, myorelaxant, anti-stress.	Basil, Bergamot, Camomile, Ginger, Peppermint, Rosemary, Lemon Verbena.	Basil, Ginger, Peppermint and Rosemary should not be used during pregnancy. Bergamot increases photosensitivity.	Localized aromatic massage in the affected area of the lower abdomen. Aromatic baths.
Flatulence	Excessive amount of air in the stomach causing the expulsion of gases either by 'burning' or 'passing wind'. The condition can occur when people are stressed, as a result of eating their food too fast or by bacterial fermentation of their food. Relaxation and close control of diet will help diminish flatulence.	Carminative, digestive, spasmolytic, laxative.	Cinnamon, Ginger, Fennel, Juniper, Lemon Grass, Thyme.	All these oils except Lemon Grass are not to be used during pregnancy and should be avoided by people who suffer from high blood pressure.	Localized aromatic massage in the affected area of the lower abdomen. Aromatic baths.

Ailments of the Digestive System *continued*

List of Ailments	Definition	Therapeutic Guide	Choice of Essential Oils	Contra-Indications and Cautions	Treatment
Halitosis	Bad breath resulting from causes such as poor oral hygiene, gum/tooth infections, infections of the lungs or sinuses or even foods such as garlic. Halitosis may also indicate a more serious problem such as the scent of ammonia in cases of kidney damage or the propanone-like scent in cases of poorly controlled diabetes.	Deodorant, antiseptic, anti-bacterial, stomachic.	**Aniseed, Fennel,** Lemon, **Peppermint.**	Aniseed, Fennel and Peppermint should not be used during pregnancy. Lemon increases photosensitivity.	**Inhalation.** Prepare a **mouth gargle:** Mix 10ml of 45° drinking spirit (Vodka or Brandy) with six drops of essential oils. Add ten drops of this mixture to a cup of boiled water and gargle regularly.
Hangover	The state of general distress experienced on the morning after an evening of alcoholic over-indulgence.	Detoxicant, excretory.	Lemon, **Peppermint, Rosemary.**	Lemon increases photosensitivity and Peppermint and Rosemary should both be avoided during pregnancy and in cases of high blood pressure.	**Inhalation.** The oils are not to be used all together, only one at a time.
Irritable Bowel Syndrome	Persistent disorder characterized by recurrent abdominal pain, flatulence, distension in the stomach and periods of diarrhoea and constipation.	Antiseptic, spasmolytic, anti-bacterial, anti-inflammatory, myorelaxants, anti-stress.	Camomile, **Cinnamon,** Lemon, Lime, **Peppermint,** Petitgrain, **Thyme.**	Cinnamon, Peppermint and Thyme are not to be used during pregnancy or where there is high blood pressure.	Daily localized **aromatic massage** in the affected area of the lower abdomen. **Aromatic baths.**

| Peptic Ulcers | Ulcer of the stomach or duodenum where there is contact with pepsin-acid gastric juice. | Antiseptic, spasmolytic, anti-bacterial, anti-inflammatory, myorelaxants, anti-stress. | Camomile, Geranium, Lavender, **Lemon Grass, Marjoram, Melissa**, Petitgrain, Lemon Verbena. | None. | **Localized aromatic massage** in the affected area of the lower abdomen. **Aromatic baths** and **inhalation**. |

Ailments of the Endocrine System

List of Ailments	*Definition*	*Therapeutic Guide*	*Choice of Essential Oils*	*Contra-Indications and Cautions*	*Treatment*
Diabetes Mellitus	Diabetes Mellitus is caused by a shortage of insulin, the hormone responsible for breaking down glucose. Diabetes tends to run in families and can occur early in life: Juvenile-onset diabetes, where the sufferers are 100% dependent on daily insulin injections. Insulin-dependent diabetics can have strong reactions to an Aromatherapy treatment and only the lightest oils and massage should be used. Diabetes Mellitus can also occur in later life and is usually controlled by diet and special tablets. This type of diabetes can be treated with Aromatherapy.	Depuratives, gentle excretory, pancreatic hormone stimulants.	Camomile, **Geranium,** Lemon **Verbena,** Pine, Ylang-Ylang.	Lemon is a photosensitive oil.	**Aromatic baths** and **massage**.

151

Ailments of the Endocrine System *continued*

List of Ailments	Definition	Therapeutic Guide	Choice of Essential Oils	Contra-Indications and Cautions	Treatment
Hyper-thyroidism	Excessive secretion of the thyroid hormone, which often affects women more than men. The condition can be worsened by stress, hot weather or an infection. It causes excessive sweating, aversion to heat, thirst, weight loss, palpitations and shortness of breath and trembling of the hands, high anxiety and emotional instability. This condition should be under medical supervision.	Anxiolytics, nerve and muscle relaxants, sedatives, metabolic retardants.	Camomile (German), **Clary Sage,** Geranium, Lavender, Lemon Verbena, Mandarin, Myrrh, Petitgrain, Vetivert.	Clary Sage should not be used during pregnancy.	**Vaporization, relaxing aromatic massage.**
Hypo-thyroidism	Deficiency of the thyroid hormone within the blood-stream. The symptoms are undue tiredness, a feeling of weakness, a hoarse voice, unusual weight gain, constipation, impaired memory, hair loss. It affects the skin and diminishes its sweating ability. This condition should be under medical supervision.	Stimulants for stamina and metabolism, sudorific, lymphotonic, nervous tonic, carminative.	Angelica, **Aniseed, Fennel, Juniper,** Niaouli.	Angelica, Aniseed, Fennel and Juniper should all be avoided during pregnancy and where there is a high blood pressure condition.	**Lymphatic massage** with essential oils is highly recommended. **Aromatic baths.**

Infertility Due to a Hormonal Imbalance	Inability to conceive which could be due to a hormonal imbalance or other problems.	Reproductive hormone balancers and stimulants.	Angelica, **Aniseed**, **Clary Sage**, Cypress, **Fennel**.	If pregnancy occurs, the treatment with these oils should cease immediately. Please note that in most circumstances, it is best to find out the medical causes of infertility before treatment.	**Deep tissue aromatic massage** and **aromatic Baths. Localized daily massage** on abdomen.

Ailments of the Excretory System

List of Ailments	Definition	Therapeutic Guide	Choice of Essential Oils	Contra-Indications and Cautions	Treatment
Candidiasis	Infection with the common yeast-like fungus of the genus *Candida*.	Fungicidal, anti-inflammatory, antiseptic, cooling, soothing.	**Cinnamon**, Niaouli, Rosewood, **Thyme**, Tea Tree.	Cinnamon and Thyme should not be used where there is high blood pressure or during pregnancy.	A special diet will be recommended under medical guidance. Localized aromatic massage of the abdominal area.
Constipation	Infrequent and difficult evacuation of the bowels.	Laxatives, carminative, nerve and muscle relaxants, depuratives.	**Cinnamon, Clary Sage, Fennel, Ginger, Juniper, Lemon Grass,** Mandarin, Orange, Petitgrain.	Cinnamon and Ginger should not be used where there is high blood pressure and Cinnamon, Clary Sage, Fennel, Ginger and Juniper should be avoided during pregnancy.	A daily **abdominal massage** in a clockwise motion.

Ailments of the Excretory System *continued*

List of Ailments	Definition	Therapeutic Guide	Choice of Essential Oils	Contra-Indications and Cautions	Treatment
Cystitis	Inflammation of the urethra and the bladder caused by bacterial infection. It is characterized by lower abdominal pain, frequent desire to pass urine, painful urination.	Anti-inflammatory, anti-bacterial, analgesic, cooling.	Bergamot, Camomile, **Eucalyptus**, **Fennel**, Geranium, Niaouli, Pine, Tea Tree, Sandalwood.	Fennel should not be used during pregnancy and Bergamot increases photosensitivity.	Depending on the acuteness, choose the least or the most powerful essential oils. Use three oils in synergy. First application: **apply six neat drops** of oil onto the skin of the lower abdominal area, above the bladder. Follow this with a course of **Sitz baths.**
Thrush	*Candida albicans* can affect the intestinal tract or the vaginal passage.	Fungicidal, anti-inflammatory, anti-bacterial, cooling, soothing.	Rosemary, Tea Tree, **Thyme**.	Rosemary and Thyme should not be used in pregnancy or in cases where there is high blood pressure.	Use the three oils in synergy blended in a carrier oil and **massage the abdomen** three times a day.

Ailments of the Immune System

List of Ailments	Definition	Therapeutic Guide	Choice of Essential Oils	Contra-Indications and Cautions	Treatment
Glandular Fever	An acute viral infection that mostly affects the ten to thirty-five years age group which often goes unrecognized. The symptoms are enlarged lymph nodes around the neck, loss of appetite, intermittent high fevers, aches and pains and a sore throat.	Anti-pyretics, anti-virals, analgesics, appetizers, immuno-stimulants.	**Cinnamon, Frankincense,** Lavender, Niaouli, Tea Tree, **Thyme.**	Cinnamon and Thyme should not be used during pregnancy and Thyme should be avoided if there is high blood pressure.	**Inhalation** and **application** of diluted essential oils onto the lymph nodes of the neck and upper chest.

Ailments of the Integumentary System

List of Ailments	Definition	Therapeutic Guide	Choice of Essential Oils	Contra-Indications and Cautions	Treatment
Abscess	Acute inflammation with the accumulation of pus in the cavity. Most often caused by bacterial infection.	Antiseptic, anti-inflammatory, antibiotic.	Cypress, **Juniper,** Lemon, Niaouli.	None because only used locally.	**Hot compress.**
Acne Vulgaris	A common disorder where there is an excessive excretion of sebum from the sebaceous glands of the skin, blocking the pores and causing bacterial infection. Can be mild or severe.	Anti-bacterial, astringent, antiseptic, anti-inflammatory anti-sebaceous.	Benzoin, Bergamot, Cypress, Geranium, **Juniper,** Lavender, **Lemon Grass,** Pine, Tea Tree, **Thyme,**	Bergamot: photo-sensitivity; Cypress, Juniper and Thyme are not to be used during pregnancy. Juniper and Thyme should not be used if	**Warm compresses. Prepare a cream** made to the following specification: blend 30g of calendula cream with twelve drops

Ailments of the Integumentary System *continued*

List of Ailments	Definition	Therapeutic Guide	Choice of Essential Oils	Contra-Indications and Cautions	Treatment
Acne Vulgaris *Continued...*	Acne occurs mostly on the face and upper back.		Ylang-Ylang.	the patient suffers from high blood pressure.	in total of Bergamot, Geranium and Tea Tree and apply three to four times per day. If this doesn't remedy the problem, then prepare a blend of the other oils and apply similarly.
Allergy	Excessive body immune response caused by acute sensitivity to allergens, bacteria and viruses.	Anti-histamine, anti-allergic, anti-inflammatory, calmative.	Respiratory: Lavender, Melissa. Digestive: Camomile, Verbena. Skin: Camomile, Geranium, Sandalwood.	None.	**Inhalations and local massage.**
Alopecia (Baldness)	Common baldness caused by a number of factors but which affects men particularly. Can be temporary, such as when caused by an infectious disease of the scalp. Permanent alopecia is more likely to be hereditary or caused by aging.	Circulatory, remedies which increase capillary circulation to the scalp.	Cedarwood, Cypress, Coriander, Myrtle, **Peppermint, Rosemary,** Ylang-Ylang.	Peppermint and Rosemary are not to be used during pregnancy; Rosemary should not be used if the patient suffers from high blood pressure.	Mix 50ml of Orange distilled water with 10ml of balsamic vinegar; add 30ml of Jojoba and 20ml of virgin olive oil plus thirty drops of essential oils. Shake well before each use and **apply in friction to the scalp only.**

	Description	Properties	Oils	Cautions	Treatment
Athlete's Foot	A fungal infection between the toes which causes the skin to become red, itchy and peeling.	Fungicide, anti-inflammatory, analgesic.	Cedarwood, Coriander, Cypress, Geranium, Grapefruit, Mandarin, Myrrh, **Rosemary, Thyme,** Tea Tree, Ylang-Ylang.	Cypress, Rosemary and Thyme are not to be used during pregnancy. Grapefruit and Mandarin also increase photosensitivity.	First prepare a **foot bath** with 50% vinegar and 50% water. After drying, **apply a cream** made to the following specifications: 30g of aqueous base cream with a total of fifteen drops of anti-fungal essential oils.
Bacterial Infection	A common bacterium today is MRSA. It is particularly found in hospitals and is creating havoc in surgical wards. MRSA is one of the hardest bacteria to treat.	Best remedies are essential oils with a high phenol content.	Oils to be used in synergy: **Eucalyptus,** Lemon, Niaouli, **Peppermint, Thyme.**	Thyme should not be used where there is a high blood pressure. Eucalyptus is not recommended in people who have a kidney disease.	**Hot compresses** applied regularly throughout the day. The oils should also be applied, blended, in a Calendula **ointment** and covered with a sterile surgical dressing.
Bed Sores	Ulcers of the skin caused by local deprivation of the blood supply as a result of the sustained pressure of lying immobile in bed for long periods.	Balsamic, cicatrisant, antiseptic, vulnerary.	Benzoin, Camomile, Geranium, **Juniper,** Lavender, Myrrh, Niaouli.	Benzoin increases photosensitivity.	Use a **compress** with Juniper and then apply a blended **ointment** made to the following specification: 30g of Calendula ointment blended with a total of fifteen drops of essential oils.

THERAPEUTIC GUIDE TO ESSENTIAL OILS

Ailments of the Integumentary System *continued*

List of Ailments	Definition	Therapeutic Guide	Choice of Essential Oils	Contra-Indications and Cautions	Treatment
Blisters caused by Friction	A type of burn to the outer layer of the skin caused by repeated friction. The sub-layer of skin fills with interstitial fluid and causes swelling.	Anaesthetic, emollients, antiseptic and cicatrisant.	Benzoin, Geranium, Lavender, Myrrh, Palmarosa.	Benzoin increases photosensitivity.	If the blister has been bleeding, it must be **washed with boiled water** before applying essential oils blended in a **Calendula ointment** and then covered lightly with a sterile gauze.
Boils and Carbuncles	Painful red swelling in the skin caused by bacterial infection of the hair follicle or sweat gland.	Anti-bacterial, astringent, antiseptic, anti-inflammatory, anti sebaceous.	**Eucalyptus, Juniper,** Pine, Tea Tree.	Juniper should not be used during pregnancy.	**Hot compress** using any of the listed oils.
Bruises	A leakage of blood from the capillaries under the skin, giving the local area a dark blue appearance.	Haemostatics, vasodilator.	Camomile, Cypress, **Juniper,** Lavender, **Marjoram.**	Cypress and Juniper should not be used during pregnancy.	Arnica **ointment** mixed with essential oils. Apply lightly to the bruised area.
Burns	A burn is tissue damage and cell death caused by exposure to intense heat, electricity, the sun (UV) or corrosive chemicals.	Antiseptic, cicatrisant, analgesic.	Lavender.	None.	After putting the burnt area of skin under running cold water, as recommended in first aid, **apply neat** Lavender

Condition	Description	Properties	Oils	Notes	Method
					and if necessary, saturate a sterile gauze with Lavender and hold it in place over the area. Further treatment: apply pure **Aloe Vera** gel mixed with 10 drops of Lavender.
Chemical Burns	Burns caused by contact with corrosive chemicals must be treated by a medical doctor.				
Contact Dermatitis	An allergic reaction caused by direct contact with certain chemicals (e.g. detergents). Causes blisters, redness, itchiness and skin damage.	Anti-inflammatory, anaesthetic, cicatrisant and vulnerary.	Benzoin, **Camomile**, **Geranium**, Myrtle, Neroli, Rose.	None.	Apply a blended ointment made to the following specifications, daily: 30g **Hypericum ointment** blended with fifteen drops of essential oils.
Cuts	Laceration of the skin.	Antiseptic, haemostatic, cicatrisant.	Lavender, Tea Tree.	None.	Initially **apply neat** Tea Tree essential oil. Apply a blend made to the following recipe: 30g Calendula ointment with fifteen drops of oil daily.
Dry Skin Condition	Excessively dry skin.	Moisturizing, emollients.	**Benzoin**, German Camomile, **Geranium**, Palmarosa, Rosewood, Rose, **Sandalwood**.	Benzoin increases photosensitivity.	**Apply aromatic oil blend** daily.

Ailments of the Integumentary System *continued*

List of Ailments	Definition	Therapeutic Guide	Choice of Essential Oils	Contra-Indications and Cautions	Treatment
Eczema	A non-infectious inflammatory disorder of the skin that can cause redness, scaling, blistering and scars. Eczema can be of psychosomatic origin or a type of allergic reaction to certain substances. Once the skin has become sensitized, it can be difficult to redress.	Anti-inflammatory, emollient, cicatrisant, moisturizing.	Benzoin, German Camomile, Geranium, Lavender, Neroli, Palmarosa, Rose, Sandalwood.	Benzoin increases photosensitivity.	Blend 50% aqueous base cream and Aloe Vera gel with twenty drops of Avocado oil and three to four drops of essential oils. **Apply** regularly.
Gingivitis	Inflammation of the gums causing pain and often minor bleeding. Can be caused by tooth decay, debilitating diseases and vitamin deficiency. Gingivitis can also be hereditary and caused by old age.	Antiseptic, anti-bacterial, anti-inflammatory, regenerative.	**Fennel**, Myrrh, Tea Tree.	Fennel is a powerful oil which should be used sparingly. It should not be used in pregnancy.	Make a mixture of 10ml of Vodka or Malt Whisky (45° alcohol) with two drops of each essential oil (total of six drops) and shake until dissolved. Then take ten drops of the above mixture to a cup of boiled water and gargle daily.
Herpes Simplex (Cold Sores)	Caused by the virus Herpes Simplex 1, painful blisters around the nose and lips	Antiseptic, anti-infectious and anti-viral and cicatrisant.	Myrrh, Rose, Tea Tree.	None.	If acute, on first application, **apply neat** Tea Tree oil.

THERAPEUTIC GUIDE TO ESSENTIAL OILS

	Description	Properties	Oils	Notes	Application
	which appear as a result of the body being depleted or after high fever or exposure to the sun.				Mix 20g of Aloe Vera gel with one drop of each of the listed oils and apply regularly.
Impetigo	A highly contagious bacterial skin infection which occurs around the mouth and nose. Appears as raised, water-filled skin lesions, and can be very itchy and irritable. It must be treated immediately.	Antiseptic, anti-viral, antibiotic.	Benzoin, Geranium, Tea Tree.	Benzoin increases photosensitivity.	Sterile gloves must be worn when handling the area. Mix 50% aqueous base cream and Aloe Vera gel and three to four drops of essential oils. **Apply** regularly.
Mouth Ulcers	Damage to the surface layer of the mucous membrane, causing pain and sometimes infection. Often the result of dietary and digestive problems.	Antiseptic, anti-bacterial, anti-inflammatory.	**Fennel**, Myrrh, Tea Tree.	Fennel is a powerful oil which should be used sparingly. It should not be used in pregnancy.	Mix 10ml of Vodka or Malt Whisky (45° alcohol) with two drops of each essential oil (total of six drops) and shake until dissolved. Then add ten drops of the above to a cup of boiled water, add half a teaspoon of bicarbonate of soda and **gargle** daily.

Ailments of the Integumentary System *continued*

List of Ailments	Definition	Therapeutic Guide	Choice of Essential Oils	Contra-Indications and Cautions	Treatment
Oily Skin	Increased production of sebum in the skin.	Astringents, anti-sebaceous	Any of the citruses, Pine, **Rosemary**, Ylang-Ylang.	Rosemary should not be used in cases of high blood pressure.	A **gentle face steam** with two to three drops of the oil (five drops maximum) in a bowl of warm water.
Psoriasis	Chronic skin condition, appears as raised patches of red and dry skin with silvery scales. Its cause is unknown but attacks are known to be triggered by trauma, infection, hormonal changes and stress. When severe, it can be disfiguring.	Anti-inflammatory, anaesthetic, cicatrisant, cooling.	Camomile (German), **Clary Sage, Juniper,** Lavender, Melissa, Rose, Sandalwood.	Clary Sage and Juniper should not be used during pregnancy.	Mix 50g of Aloe Vera gel with 50g of aqueous base cream and then add 10g of Calendula cream. To this mixture, blend thirty drops of essential oils and **apply** regularly to the body.
Rashes	Skin irritation showing red patches or spotty skin, sometimes very itchy. Can be caused by exposure to dampness (wet nappies), can be a sign of a communicable disease (measles) or a sign of skin infection caused by bacteria or fungus.	Anti-inflammatory, cooling, emollient.	Benzoin, Camomile (Roman), Geranium, Lavender, Sandalwood.	Benzoin increases photosensitivity.	Apply a **cold compress** (use cooled boiled water). Afterwards apply Aloe Vera gel blended with two or three of the essential oils as often as needed.

Ringworm	A fungal infection that affects the keratinized portion of the skin, hair or nails and produces circular patchy scaling and inflammation.	Fungicide, anti-inflammatory, analgesic.	**Eucalyptus,** Cypress, **Lemon Grass,** Tea Tree.	Cypress should not be used during pregnancy.	**Neat applications** starting with Tea Tree. If this is not successful then use in synergy with Cypress, Eucalyptus and if necessary Lemon Grass.
Scleroderma	Thickening and hardening of the skin giving smooth, shiny and tight appearance. It can shrink areas of skin and hinder some movements. It is known to be part of a general systemic disturbance and is classified as an immune disorder. The causes of these disorders are not known. Sometimes it appears as one of the symptoms of Lupus Erythematosus.	Emollients, cytophyllactics, moisturizers, re-hydratants, rubefacient.	Camomile (German), Geranium, Neroli, Palmarosa, Rose, Rosewood, Ylang-Ylang.	None.	Blend 40ml of aqueous base lotion with 10ml of un-refined Jojoba and 10ml of unrefined Rose Hip oil. To this add fifteen drops of essential oils. **Apply** regularly.
Shingles	A disease caused by the reactivation of an early infection with chicken pox, which often has remained dormant for many years. Can be brought on by stress.	Antiseptic, anti-infectious and anti-viral, analgesic.	**Benzoin, Eucalyptus,** Niaouli, Lavender, Tea Tree.	Benzoin increases photosensitivity.	Wear surgical gloves as the pustules are highly infectious and **apply** Aloe Vera gel blended with the essential oils.

163

Ailments of the Integumentary System *continued*

List of Ailments	Definition	Therapeutic Guide	Choice of Essential Oils	Contra-Indications and Cautions	Treatment
Stings (Wasps and Bees)	The reaction caused by the sting depends on individual sensitivity and the variety of insect. For most people it will cause redness, swelling, itchiness and pain. Occasionally, in an individual with an allergy to them, it can cause a potentially lethal reaction, such as anaphylactic shock where all body systems collapse. This must be treated immediately by a medical doctor.	Anti-inflammatory, anti-poison, anti-histamine, analgesic.	**Peppermint**, Lavender.	Peppermint should not be used in pregnancy.	**Neat oil** to be applied directly to the sting. On children over two, add two drops of Peppermint to 10ml of balsamic vinegar and apply to the affected area.
Sunburn	The damaging effect of the ultraviolet component of sunlight on the skin can cause redness and severe blistering. Although simple sunburn does not require much treatment, severe sunburn may require medical advice.	Cooling, moisturizing, soothing, analgesic.	Lavender, Tea Tree.	None.	Blend Aloe Vera gel with the essential oils and **apply** to the area.
Ulcers of the Skin	The temporary loss of the upper epithelium or mucous membrane, leaving the layer below exposed to dehydration, infection and further damage. Can be	Antiseptic, anti-inflammatory, cicatrisant, analgesic, emollients.	Benzoin, Camomile (Roman), Cypress, Geranium, Lavender, Myrrh, Palmarosa, Tea Tree.	Benzoin increases photosensitivity and Cypress should be avoided during pregnancy.	**Calendula ointment** blended with essential oils. Apply regularly.

Condition	Description	Properties	Oils	Cautions	Application
	painful and is often caused by damage to the skin by heat or cold, continued pressure, waterlogged tissues and poor blood supply to the area.				
Urticaria (Hives)	A skin eruption which looks similar to nettle rash, causing intense itchiness. It is an allergic reaction caused by emotional stress, anxiety or sensitivity to some foods or chemicals. It can run in families and is fairly common in children.	Anti-inflammatory, cooling, emollient, analgesic.	Cedarwood, Lavender, Melissa, Sandalwood.	None.	**Aloe Vera gel mixed with the essential oils.**
Verruca/Wart	A small, solid, benign tumour that arises from the surface of the skin and is caused by a viral infection. They are extremely common and harmless but are nevertheless infectious. Can be painful.	Anti-viral.	Cypress, Lemon, Tea Tree.	Cypress should not be used during pregnancy.	**Neat application.**
Wounds	An injury involving a break in the surface of the skin or an organ.	Antiseptic, anti-infectious, cicatrisant, anti-inflammatory, vulnerary.	**Eucalyptus, Frankincense,** Geranium, **Juniper,** Lavender, Lemon, Pine, Tea Tree.	Thyme and Juniper should not be used in pregnancy, Lemon increases photo-sensitivity and Thyme should not be used on people with high blood pressure. Juniper is not to be used where there is kidney disease.	**Hot compresses** applied regularly throughout the day. The oils should also be applied, blended in a **Calendula ointment** and then covered with a sterile surgical dressing.

Ailments of the Lymphatic System

List of Ailments	Definition	Therapeutic Guide	Choice of Essential Oils	Contra-Indications and Cautions	Treatment
Cellulite	Necrosis of some of the adipose tissue cells in the subcutaneous tissue with mild accumulation of interstitial fluid causing the skin to look like an orange peel. Can appear at puberty or later on with weight gains. Mostly shows on the limbs and abdomen.	Sudorific, lymphotonic, lymph decongestant, venous decongestant, diuretic.	Cedarwood, **Clary Sage**, Cypress, **Fennel**, Geranium, Grapefruit, **Juniper**, Lemon, Lime, Myrtle, Palmarosa, Pine, **Rosemary, Thyme.**	Cedarwood, Clary Sage, Cypress, Fennel, Juniper, Rosemary and Thyme should not be used during pregnancy. Clary Sage and Cypress should not be used on people who have mastitis. Fennel, Pine, Rosemary and Thyme should not be used on people with high blood pressure. Grapefruit, Lemon and Lime increase photosensitivity.	**Lymphatic massage,** application to the body of an aromatic blend with the use of a **steam room. Aromatic baths, skin-brushing and exercise.**
Obesity	Excessive body weight with fluid retention, can be caused by an endocrine disorder, illnesses, through self-indulgent lifestyle or can be hereditary.	Diuretic, sudorific, lymph decongestant, hepatic tonic, expectorant.	Angelica, **Basil,** Camomile, **Fennel,** Geranium, Ginger, Grapefruit, **Juniper,** Lemon, Myrtle, Pine, **Rosemary, Thyme.**	Angelica, Basil, Fennel, Ginger, Juniper, Pine, Rosemary and Thyme should not be used during pregnancy. Ginger, Pine, Rosemary, and Thyme should not be used where there is a high blood pressure condition. Angelica, Grapefruit and Lemon increase photosensitivity.	To lose weight safely, it is important first to have a **medical check-up** and to have a realistic aim so as not to endanger other vital organs. **Lymphatic massage, specialized diet** and monitored **exercise.**

List of Ailments	Definition	Therapeutic Guide	Choice of Essential Oils	Contra-Indications and Cautions	Treatment
Water Retention	Can be caused by minor or major vascular problems such as poor circulation or high blood pressure but often it is caused by poor re-absorption of fluid by the lymphatic system. Each individual's lymphatic system has a variable ability to re-absorb tissue fluid, particularly in the limbs and abdomen. This condition is especially common in the over-forty age group.	Lymph decongestant, venous decongestant, vasoconstrictor, sudorific, diuretic.	Clary Sage, Geranium, Grapefruit, Myrtle, Palmarosa, **Pine**, **Rosemary**, Sandalwood.	Clary Sage, Pine and Rosemary should not be used during pregnancy. Pine and Rosemary should not be used when there is a high blood pressure condition. Grapefruit increases photo-sensitivity.	Apply aromatic blend daily before bath. **Lymphatic massage and gentle exercise.**

Ailments of the Muscular System

List of Ailments	*Definition*	*Therapeutic Guide*	*Choice of Essential Oils*	*Contra-Indications and Cautions*	*Treatment*
Atrophy	A wasting or decrease in the size of a muscle which prevents its use.	Vasodilator, cytophyllactics, peripheral nerves stimulant.	**Aniseed, Basil, Cinnamon,** Geranium, Lemon, Marjoram, Pine, **Rosemary.**	Aniseed, Basil, Cinnamon, Pine and Rosemary are not to be used during pregnancy. Basil, Cinnamon, Pine and Rosemary should not be used where there is a high blood pressure condition. Lemon increases photosensitivity.	**Localized daily massage** and **aromatic baths.**

Ailments of the Muscular System *continued*

List of Ailments	Definition	Therapeutic Guide	Choice of Essential Oils	Contra-Indications and Cautions	Treatment
Frozen Shoulder	Painful, persistent stiffness of the shoulder joint that restricts normal movement. Sometimes leads to severe inflammation of the joint.	Anti-spasmodics, myorelaxants, analgesics, vasodilators, anti-inflammatories.	**Basil, Black Pepper,** Camomile, **Cinnamon, Clary Sage,** Ginger, Lavender, **Marjoram, Peppermint,** Pine, **Rosemary,** Lemon Verbena.	Basil, Black Pepper, Cinnamon, Clary Sage, Ginger, Peppermint, Pine and Rosemary should not be used during pregnancy. Basil, Black Pepper, Cinnamon, Ginger and Rosemary should not be used where there is a high blood pressure condition. Lemon increases photosensitivity.	**Aromatic oil application** daily combined with **Swedish massage** of the neck, back and both shoulders. **Hot aromatic baths** or **hot compresses.**
Muscle Spasm	Painful involuntary contraction of one or more muscles. Can be caused by postural defects, an injury while in motion, colds and flu or muscle fibre inflammation due to the accumulation of lactic acid.	Spasmolytics, myorelaxants, anti-inflammatories, analgesics, lymphotonics, circulatory stimulants, nerve relaxants.	**Aniseed, Basil,** Camomile, **Cinnamon, Clary Sage,** Fennel, **Ginger,** Lavender, Lemon, **Marjoram,** Peppermint, **Rosemary,** Ylang-Ylang.	Aniseed, Basil, Cinnamon, Clary Sage, Fennel, Ginger, Peppermint and Rosemary are not to be used during pregnancy. Cinnamon, Ginger and Rosemary should not be used where there is a high blood pressure condition. Lemon increases photosensitivity.	**Aromatic Swedish massage, hot aromatic baths.**

Condition	Description	Properties	Oils	Cautions	Application
Muscle Stiffness (from Over-exercising)	Can be due to an excess of lactic acid deposited in the skeletal muscles.	Analgesic, myorelaxant, lymph decongestant, anti-inflammatory, lymphotonic.	Camomile, **Cinnamon, Clary Sage**, Lavender, **Marjoram**, Pine, **Rosemary, Thyme.**	Cinnamon, Clary Sage, Rosemary and Thyme should not be used during pregnancy. Cinnamon, Rosemary and Thyme should not be used where there is a high blood pressure condition.	**Daily aromatic oil application** combined with **Swedish massage. Hot aromatic baths, hot compresses.**
Muscular Cramps	Abnormally sustained and usually powerful contraction of the muscle.	Analgesic, myorelaxant, warming, anti-inflammatory, nerve relaxant.	Camomile (Roman), **Clary Sage**, Lavender, **Marjoram**, Pine, **Rosemary, Thyme.**	Clary Sage, Rosemary and Thyme should not be used during pregnancy. Rosemary and Thyme should not be used where there is a high blood pressure condition.	**Gentle aromatic massage** and **aromatic baths.**
Muscular Dystrophy	Mostly a hereditary disorder, for which there is no known cure, muscular dystrophy leads to chronic muscular fatigue due to a degeneration of the muscles.	Neuro-muscular stimulant, anti-spasmodic, analgesic.	**Basil**, Camomile, **Clary Sage,** Lavender, **Marjoram,** Lemon, Lemon Grass, Lemon Verbena and **Rosemary.**	Basil, Clary Sage and Rosemary should not be used during pregnancy. Rosemary should not be used where there is a high blood pressure condition. Lemon increases photosensitivity.	Regular **gentle massage** of the affected area.
Myalgia	Muscular pain.	Analgesics, myorelaxant.	**Black Pepper,** Camomile, Lavender, **Marjoram.**	Black Pepper should not be used during pregnancy or on anyone with high blood pressure.	**Localized massage application.**

Ailments of the Muscular System *continued*

List of Ailments	Definition	Therapeutic Guide	Choice of Essential Oils	Contra-Indications and Cautions	Treatment
Rheumatism	Common term for pain and stiffness in joints and muscles, as well as for major disorders such as rheumatoid arthritis.	Anti-inflammatory, analgesic, anti-spasmodic, excretory.	**Black Pepper,** Camomile, **Cinnamon,** Ginger, Juniper, Lavender, Marjoram, Pine, **Rosemary.**	Black Pepper, Cinnamon, Ginger, Juniper and Rosemary should not be used during pregnancy. Black Pepper, Ginger and Rosemary should not be used on anyone with high blood pressure.	**Localized massage, aromatic massage** and **baths.**
Sprain	Sprain or partial tear in the ligaments of a joint and to the adjacent tissues caused by injuries or a fall. Slow to mend and very painful, e.g. sprained ankle.	Anti-inflammatory, anti-spasmodic, anti-oedematous, analgesic.	**Cypress,** Geranium, **Juniper,** Lavender, **Marjoram.**	Cypress and Juniper should not be used during pregnancy and Cypress should be avoided by people with a high blood pressure condition.	**Ice-pack** to decrease the swelling, **cold aromatic compresses** and later on apply **Arnica ointment** with essential oils regularly.
Tendonitis	Inflammation of muscular tendons which can be painful. Carpal Tunnel Syndrome, found in persons who use their hands and fingers a lot. Prevents the full use of the hand.	Anti-inflammatory, analgesic, cytophylactic.	Camomile, Geranium, Lavender, Pine, **Rosemary, Thyme.**	Rosemary and Thyme should be avoided during pregnancy and by people with high blood pressure.	**Arnica ointment** blended with the essential oils applied as often as needed. If acute, may need bandaging.

Ailments of the Nervous System

List of Ailments	Definition	Therapeutic Guide	Choice of Essential Oils	Contra-Indications and Cautions	Treatment
Anorexia Nervosa	Loss of appetite: serious disorder of perception where a person is exercising voluntary dietary restriction over a period of time to improve figure. It leads to emaciation causing the sufferer to drastically lose a great deal of weight and become emaciated. Mostly affects teenage girls but these days also older women and young men.	Myorelaxants, anti-depressants, appetizers.	**Aniseed,** Angelica, Camomile, Citruses, Jasmine, Melissa.	Aniseed is not for people suffering from hallucinations and delirium. Angelica is an emmenagogue and photosensitizer.	**Vaporizations:** Aniseed and Lemon or Jasmine to uplift the mood. **Aromatic massage** and **bath:** Citrus oils and Melissa for hysteria and over-exertion; Angelica: to restore hormonal balance; Camomile: to regulate digestive spasms.
Anxiety	This is a normal response to a crisis (driving test, etc.), but when it is excessive and prolonged it can become socially crippling. It can lead to obsessive behaviour and it is an important factor in depressive states. The symptoms include headaches, loss of appetite and weight, palpitations, disrupted sleep, fear, sweating and sudden tearful outbursts.	Hypnotics, myorelaxants, calmatives.	**Clary Sage, Frankincense,** Mandarin, Melissa, Neroli, Patchouli, Petitgrain, Ylang-Ylang.	Not recommended for people with excessively low blood pressure.	Vaporization, inhalations, **aromatic massage and bath.**

Ailments of the Nervous System *continued*

List of Ailments	Definition	Therapeutic Guide	Choice of Essential Oils	Contra-Indications and Cautions	Treatment
Depression	Persistent unhappy mood with symptoms such as low energy, loss of appetite, poor concentration, insomnia, guilt, loss of libido and inability to partake in social activities. This condition can be temporary or chronic; the former is caused by sudden traumatic events, while the condition and does not always latter is a more prolonged have known causes. It is the modern term for melancholy.	Anti-depressants, relaxants, sedatives and tonics.	**Basil**, Bergamot, **Frankincense**, **Fennel**, **Geranium**, Grapefruit, Lavender, Melissa, Rosemary.	Basil and Frankincense: not recommended for mental agitation, anger and confusion; Fennel: not recommended for people with mood swings. Rosemary: not recommended for people with high blood pressure.	**Aromatic baths, massage, inhalations; anti-depressants** and **tonic oils**: Bergamot, Frankincense, Fennel, Grapefruit, Rosemary; **relaxants** and **sedatives**: Lavender, Melissa, Ylang-Ylang.
Drugs and Drink Abuse Recovery	The recovery phase after quitting drink or drug dependency includes detoxification and strengthening the mind through therapy.	Mood enhancers, anti-depressants, sedatives, diuretics and sudorifics.	Camomile (Roman), **Clary Sage**, Coriander, Geranium, Jasmine, **Juniper**, **Marjoram**, Lemon Verbena.	Juniper: not suitable for people with liver and kidney damage. Juniper and Clary Sage should also not be used in pregnancy.	**Vaporization:** Clary Sage and Geranium. **Aromatic massage and baths:** Clary Sage, Coriander, Geranium and Lemon Verbena, particularly indicated for mood swings and depression. Juniper: indicated for detoxifi-

Emotional and Physical Depletion	Sense of emptiness after undergoing an intense phase of stress. This can happen after caring for a dying relative or something similar.	Hypnotic, anti-depressant, nervous tonic.	Angelica, Bergamot and other citruses, **Frankincense,** Geranium, Jasmine, Neroli, Rose, Rosewood and Sandalwood.	cation. Camomile and Marjoram: indicated for insomnia. Angelica and Neroli: not recommended for people who feel apathetic and Angelica is never to be used in pregnancy. Frank-incense: not recommended if suffering from 'flashbacks'.	**Vaporization, inhalations, aromatic massage and baths.**
Epilepsy	A chronic disorder involving abnormal electrical discharge in the brain. It causes seizures and can result in a loss of consciousness. The cause is unknown, but tumours can interfere with brain tissue, resulting in epilepsy.	Hypnotics, mental relaxants, calmatives and sedatives.	Camomile, Lavender, Mandarin, Neroli, Rose, Vetivert and Ylang-Ylang.	None.	**Vaporization, inhalation and aromatic massage.** The essential oils found to be most useful for epilepsy are Jasmine, Neroli, Rose and Ylang-Ylang.
Fatigue	Extreme physical and mental tiredness.	Nervous tonics and relaxants.	Geranium, Grapefruit, Ginger, Lavender, Lime, Pine, Lemon Verbena and Ylang-Ylang.	Ginger: not to be used in cases of high blood pressure or pregnancy.	**Aromatic massage and baths.** The best oils for day-time usage are: citruses, Ginger, Pine and Lemon Verbena. The best oils for evening use are: Geranium, Lavender and Ylang-Ylang.

Ailments of the Nervous System *continued*

List of Ailments	Definition	Therapeutic Guide	Choice of Essential Oils	Contra-Indications and Cautions	Treatment
Fear	The natural response by the autonomic nervous system to real or imagined dangers. Symptoms are panic, palpitations, inability to move, extreme anger, inability to speak or other impaired functions, sweating, colic and sometimes unspecified areas of pain.	Anxiolytics, myorelaxants, spasmolytics.	Bergamot, Geranium, **Marjoram**, Melissa, Orange, Petitgrain, Rosewood, Vetivert, Ylang-Ylang.	Bergamot is a photosensitive oil.	**Vaporization and aromatic baths.**
Frigidity	Lack of sexual desire in a woman or failure to respond in sexual intercourse. It can be caused by poor general health, depression or can be of psychological origins.	Anxiolytics, myorelaxants, aphrodisiacs.	Cinnamon, **Clary Sage**, Coriander, Frankincense, **Jasmine**, Patchouli, **Rosewood**, Sandalwood, Ylang-Ylang.	Cinnamon is not to be used in cases of high blood pressure.	**Vaporization, inhalation and aromatic massage baths.**
Hyperactivity	Intense restless condition common in children today, can be caused by certain food additives, hormone imbalance or psychological disturbance.	Calmatives, relaxants, moderators, hypnotics.	Benzoin, Lavender, **Marjoram, Melissa, Neroli**, Patchouli, Petitgrain, Lemon Verbena, Vetivert, Ylang-Ylang.	Note that dosage of oils for children should be lower than that for adults. Citruses and Lavender are better for children.	**Vaporization, aromatic baths.**
Hypochondria	A neurotic condition regarding one's general state of health, usually of psychological origins, where a person becomes obsessed with illness in the body and tends to magnify or invent health problems.	Hypnotics, mental relaxants and calmatives.	Angelica, Geranium, Mandarin, Melissa, Neroli, Petitgrain, Rose, Rosewood, Sandalwood, Vetivert, Ylang-Ylang.	Angelica is never to be used in pregnancy.	**Aromatic baths and massage.**

It is associated with mental illness and depression.

	Description		Oils		Application
Hysteria	Defined as an excessive emotional response due to traumatic events or mental illness. It is thought to be a mental response when confronted by high anxiety or life-threatening situations. The symptoms are: hyperactivity, loss of memory of certain events, hysterical fits (endless screaming), sleepwalking, paralysis, blindness, deafness, vomiting, or loss of sensation in parts of the body. It can be temporary or long term.	Calmatives, sedatives, hypnotics, nerve relaxants, anxiolytics.	Camomile, **Clary Sage, Frankincense,** Geranium, Jasmine, Lavender, Mandarin, **Marjoram, Melissa, Neroli,** Orange, Petitgrain, Rose, Violet, Ylang-Ylang.	Frankincense is not an oil for someone who lives in a fantasy world. Clary Sage should not be used during pregnancy and may slow reflexes; caution should be taken with driving.	**Vaporization, aromatic baths and massage.**
Impotence	The inability to achieve or sustain a firm penile erection to allow normal vaginal sexual intercourse. It can occur as a result of anxiety, depression, fear, preoccupation or fatigue. However, chronic debilitating diseases, alcoholism, drug addiction, diseases of the nervous system or endocrine disorders, pharmaceutical drugs and damage to the urethra can all be responsible for the condition.	Hypnotics, nervine relaxants, anxiolytics.	**Black Pepper, Cinnamon,** Coriander, Ginger, Pine, Rosewood, **Thyme,** Ylang-Ylang.	Cinnamon, Ginger and Thyme are not to be used in cases of high blood pressure.	**Vaporization, Aromatherapy treatment by professionals and aromatic baths.**

Ailments of the Nervous System *continued*

List of Ailments	Definition	Therapeutic Guide	Choice of Essential Oils	Contra-Indications and Cautions	Treatment
Insomnia	Difficulty in falling asleep or remaining asleep for an acceptable period of time. It can be caused by anxiety or depression and extreme exhaustion.	Sedatives, myorelaxants, nervine relaxants.	Angelica, Benzoin, Camomile, Cedarwood, Geranium, Lavender, Mandarin, **Marjoram**, Myrrh, Neroli, Orange, Patchouli, Petitgrain, Rose, Sandalwood, Vetivert, Ylang-Ylang.	Angelica: not to be used in pregnancy.	**Vaporization, inhalation, aromatic baths, Aromatherapy massage.**
Melancholy	Melancholy is the ancient word for depression, except that it particularly referred to deep sadness, sometimes for no known reason. Sometimes, the sadness was a characteristic in the sufferer's temperament.	The remedies should be the ones that counter sadness by bringing warmth and joy to the heart.	The traditional remedies for melancholy are Angelica, Camomile, Jasmine, Marjoram, Melissa, Rose, Rosemary, Violet.	Angelica is not to be used during pregnancy.	Any of the oils could be worn as a **personal perfume; aromatic massages** and **baths** are also recommended.
Migraine	A throbbing headache which affects only one half of the head. Symptoms are visual disturbances, blurred vision, streaks of shining light creating blind spots in the vision, localized numbness, halos around objects, severe pain in the head and sometimes nausea and vomiting. Attacks can be linked to diet and food	Nervine relaxants, myorelaxants and analgesics.	**Geranium**, Lavender, **Melissa**, Peppermint.	Peppermint is not to be used during pregnancy and can cause irritation to a sensitive skin.	**Localized massage** to the temples or the neck and shoulders. Usually the essential oils will be diluted but if acute, Lavender used neat may be suitable.

allergies. It can also be a symptom of other illnesses.

	Description	Properties	Essential Oils	Cautions	Application
Mood Swings	Quick changes of moods from states of euphoria to intense sadness. A common symptom in manic depression, it can also be caused by hormonal changes in the body at puberty, after childbirth or at the menopause and can be caused by drug and alcohol addiction.	Hypnotic and natural tranquillizers.	Bergamot, **Clary Sage**, Geranium, Jasmine, Lavender, Neroli, Rosewood, Sandalwood, Vetivert and Ylang-Ylang.	Bergamot increases photosensitivity and Clary Sage should not be used during pregnancy and may slow reflexes; caution should be taken when driving.	**Inhalation, aromatic baths** and **massage**.
Nervous Debility	Mental and emotional stress accompanied by muscular tension throughout the body. It can be caused by shyness, lack of proper relaxation or having to face too many difficult situations.	Myorelaxants and spasmolytics.	**Aniseed, Cinnamon, Clary Sage**, Geranium, Lavender, Lemon Grass, **Marjoram, Rosemary, Thyme**, Lemon Verbena.	Aniseed can induce euphoria. Clary Sage should not be used during pregnancy and may slow reflexes; caution should be taken when driving.	**Aromatic massage** and baths.
Neurasthenia	Nervous exhaustion leading to poor concentration, loss of memory and lack of physical stamina. It is a form of depression associated with severe neurosis, morbidity and phobia.	Expectorant, nervine stimulant, tonic, sudorific.	Camomile, Coriander, Frankincense, Lemon, Lemon Verbena, Marjoram, Neroli, Vetivert, Violet, Ylang-Ylang.	Basil, Frankincense and Rosemary are strong nerve stimulants.	**Inhalations, aromatic baths**.

Ailments of the Nervous System *continued*

List of Ailments	Definition	Therapeutic Guide	Choice of Essential Oils	Contra-Indications and Cautions	Treatment
Neuralgia	A pain arriving along the course of a nerve. It may be severe, dull or stabbing. It can occur anywhere on the body or on the face.	Analgesic, anaesthetic, spasmolytics, nerve relaxants, anti-inflammatory.	**Basil**, Camomile, **Clary Sage**, Geranium, Ginger, Lavender, Myrrh, Neroli, Pine, Ylang-Ylang.	Basil can overstimulate the central nervous system. Clary Sage should not be used during pregnancy and may slow reflexes. Ginger should also be avoided during pregnancy and is not suitable for those with high blood pressure.	**Localized application** where essential oils are blended in an alcoholic solution. If acute or for first aid, Lavender and Basil blended in a carrier; dosage about 8% oil, applied on the area and, if possible, near the zone of the root of the nerve.
Nightmares	Frightening dreams occurring during the lighter part of sleep: REM.	Hypnotics, natural tranquillizers and sedatives.	**Camomile**, Geranium, Lavender, **Marjoram**, Neroli, Sandalwood, Vetivert, Violet.	None.	**Vaporization, inhalation, aromatic massage and baths.**
Panic Attacks	Acute anxiety or fear which can cause distress, palpitations, hyperventilation and fainting. Most likely to occur after traumatic situations and repeated stress.	Sedatives, myorelaxants, spasmolytics, nerve relaxants.	Angelica, Camomile, Geranium, Jasmine, Lavender, **Marjoram**, Melissa, Neroli, Rose, Ylang-Ylang.	Angelicas increase photosensitivity and should be avoided during pregnancy.	**Vaporization, inhalation, aromatic baths** and **massage**.

Psychosomatic Disorders	Physical disorders of psychological origins where physical disorders have no specific or recognised cause.	Many of the disorders are caused by sensitivity to the environment or to a hyper-excitability of certain reflexes controlled by the autonomic nervous system, therefore what is often needed is a remedy that decreases sensitivity or slows down the reflex.	Camomile, Clary Sage, Citruses, Geranium, Lavender, Melissa, Neroli, **Thyme**, Ylang-Ylang.	Thyme should not be used where there is high blood pressure.	**Aromatic massages, baths** and **inhalations**.
Shock	There are different types of shock, this relates more to emotional shock. It will cause tearful states, shaking, lack of confidence, stuttering and lack of interest in one's circumstances.	Calmatives, myorelaxants, sedatives.	Angelica, Lavender, Jasmine, Melissa, Neroli, Rose, Rosewood, Ylang-Ylang.	Be careful with Angelica as it is a photosensitizer.	**Aromatic massage** and **baths**.
Stress	Constant state of pressure caused by lifestyle or specific situations, will lead to symptoms of restlessness, irritability, sleeplessness, impatience, depression, digestive disorders, muscular tensions, tiredness, impaired breathing, skin ailments or other.	Nervine and cardiac tonics, anxiolytic, nervine and myorelaxants, sedatives, calmatives, expectorant, energizers, sudorifics.	Angelica, Benzoin, Camomile, all the citruses, Coriander, Geranium, Ginger, Lavender, Neroli, Myrtle, Palmarosa, Rose, Rosewood, Ylang-Ylang.	Angelica should not be used during pregnancy and causes increased photosensitivity. Ginger should not be used in cases where there is high blood pressure or in pregnancy.	**Aromatic massage** and **baths**.

Ailments of the Nervous System *continued*

List of Ailments	Definition	Therapeutic Guide	Choice of Essential Oils	Contra-Indications and Cautions	Treatment
Trauma	Any event which has an adverse psychological effect, whether one is a witness, a participant or the direct recipient to such a situation.	Nervine relaxant, myorelaxant, sedative.	**Clary Sage,** Jasmine, Lavender, Neroli, **Frankincense,** Rose, Ylang-Ylang.	Clary Sage should not be used during pregnancy.	**Aromatic massage** and **baths.**

Ailments of the Reproductive System

List of Ailments	Definition	Therapeutic Guide	Choice of Essential Oils	Contra-Indications and Cautions	Treatment
After Giving Birth	To heal minor internal tissue damage or tears.	Analgesic, anti-inflammatory, cicatrisant, vasoconstrictor.	Benzoin, Camomile, Cypress, Geranium, Jasmine, Lavender, Myrrh, Tea Tree.	None.	For minor internal damage in the birth passage, blend two-thirds Calendula ointment to one-third Aloe Vera gel mixed with Camomile, Geranium and Lavender. To be applied internally as needed. Generally, aromatic baths with Jasmine blended with two other essential oils.

After Giving Birth	For tiredness.	Tonics, energizers and stimulating oils.	Grapefruit, Lime, Lemon Verbena, **Rosemary**, Rosewood.	Rosemary is an emmenagogue; it must not be used on anyone with a high blood pressure condition.	Full Aromatherapy treatment and aromatic baths.
After Giving Birth	For postnatal depression.	Anti-depressants, tonics, energizers, anxiolytics.	Geranium, Jasmine, Lemon, Lime, Lemon Verbena, Melissa, Rose, Rosewood, Ylang-Ylang.	Rosemary is an emmenagogue; it must not be used on anyone with a high blood pressure condition; Lemon and Lime increase photosensitivity.	Vaporizations, inhalations, aromatic massage and baths.
Amenorrhoea	The absence of a woman's period due to a possible hormonal imbalance, emotional shock, poor health, excessive weight loss or acute stress.	Emmenagogue, anti-stress.	Angelica, **Cinnamon**, **Fennel**, **Peppermint**, **Rosemary**, Thyme.	Note that these oils are highly potent and no more than two should be used at the same time.	**Lower abdominal massage and aromatic baths.**
Dysmenorrhoea	Irregular periods which could be caused by disruption to the hormonal cycle or could be the onset of an illness.	Hormone regulator, anti-stress.	Angelica, Geranium, **Fennel**, Melissa, Palmarosa, Rose, Ylang-Ylang.	Angelica and Fennel are both emmenagogues.	**Local aromatic massage.**
Mastitis	Inflammation of the breast. It often occurs when a woman begins breast-feeding and can cause fever, painful and congested breasts and abscesses. It is usually of hormonal origin.	Anti-inflammatories, analgesic, vasodilators, lymphotonics, lymph decongestant.	Camomile, Geranium, Lavender, **Marjoram**, Palmarosa, Sandalwood.	None.	Application of aromatic blend on the upper arms, upper chest and both breasts.

Ailments of the Reproductive System *continued*

List of Ailments	Definition	Therapeutic Guide	Choice of Essential Oils	Contra-Indications and Cautions	Treatment
Mastitis *continued*	Chronic mastitis refers to a cystic condition of the breast and can cause changes in the tissues such as fibrosis, hardened tissues, pain and congestion. This is also connected with the phases of the menstrual cycle.				
Menopause	Menopause in the life of a woman signals the end of her reproductive years. This is the time when oestrogen and progesterone levels fluctuate and begin to decline. Some of the changes that occur include anxiety, mood swings, depression, pessimism, hot flushes, forgetfulness, headaches, insomnia, PMS, palpitations, swollen or stiff joints.	Anxiolytics, anti-depressants, energizers, hormone regulators, mood enhancers.	Angelica, Geranium, Jasmine, Lavender, Melissa, Neroli, Palmarosa, Patchouli, Rose, Rosewood, Violet, Verbena, Ylang-Ylang.	Angelica is an emmenagogue and increases photosensitivity.	**Aromatic body lotions, aromatic massages and baths.**
Miscarriage (to Heal the Trauma)	A miscarriage often leaves a woman with a feeling of emptiness and a great fear about further pregnancies.	Restorative, beautifying.	Clary Sage, Jasmine, Mandarin, Melissa, Neroli, Rose, Rosewood, Sandalwood, Ylang-Ylang.	Clary Sage is an emmenagogue.	**Full Aromatherapy** treatment by professional Aromatherapist and **daily aromatic baths at home.**

List of Ailments	Definition	Therapeutic Guide	Choice of Essential Oils	Contra-Indications and Cautions	Treatment
Premenstrual Syndrome/ Menstruation	Physical and emotional symptoms associated with PMS: drastic mood swings, bloatedness, aches and pains, lower back ache, sore breasts and water retention.	Anxiolytic, calmative, lymph decongestant, anti-spasmodic, analgesic.	Angelica, **Clary Sage**, Geranium, Lavender, Jasmine, Melissa, Palmarosa, Petitgrain, Ylang-Ylang.	Angelica and Clary Sage are emmenagogues and Angelica increases photosensitivity.	**Aromatic massage** and **baths**.
Ailments of the Respiratory System					
Acute Chest Infections	Infections caused by viruses or bacteria which can affect one or both sides of the chest. They can cause fever, pain, breathing difficulties and excessive mucous discharge.	Antiseptic, anti-bacterial/anti-viral, balsamic, mucolytic, expectorant, anti-inflammatory, anti-spasmodic, pectoral.	Benzoin, **Black Pepper, Clary Sage, Cinnamon, Eucalyptus,** Fennel, Ginger, **Juniper,** Lavender, Myrtle, Niaouli, **Peppermint,** Pine, **Rose, Thyme.**	Black Pepper, Clary Sage, Cinnamon, Fennel, Ginger, Juniper, Peppermint and Thyme are not to be used during pregnancy. Black Pepper, Fennel, Ginger, Juniper and Thyme should be avoided by people with high blood pressure. Black Pepper is a mucous membrane irritant.	**Inhalations,** application of **aromatic oil blend** to front and back of the chest. **Keep warm.**
Asthma	A narrowing of the bronchioles, restricting the passage of air in and out of the lungs. Breathing becomes difficult and expiration is more difficult than inspiration. Shortness of breath, coughing	Broncho-dilators, balsamic, spasmolytics, anti-stressors, anti-inflammatories, nerve relaxants.	Camomile, **Frankincense,** Geranium, Lavender, Neroli, Rose, Ylang-Ylang.	None.	**Vaporization, aromatic massage,** particularly in the shoulder and chest area.

Ailments of the Respiratory System *continued*

List of Ailments	Definition	Therapeutic Guide	Choice of Essential Oils	Contra-Indications and Cautions	Treatment
Asthma *continued*	wheezing and diminished chest movement are all the symptoms. It can be caused by an allergy, prolonged exertion and emotional factors such as stress and anxiety.				
Bronchitis	An inflammation of the bronchi, characterized by enlargement of glands and goblet cells lining the bronchial airways. Can be acute or chronic, resulting in a painful cough, mild fever, aching muscles and depression, then a profuse expulsion of mucus. Acute bronchitis often follows a cold or an attack of bacterial or viral infection.	Antiseptic, anti-spasmodic, expectorant, anti-inflammatory, mucolytic, balsamic, anti-infectious.	Angelica, Benzoin, Cedarwood, **Eucalyptus,** Ginger, **Juniper,** Lavender, Myrtle, Niaouli, Pine, Tea Tree.	Angelica, Ginger and Juniper should not be used during pregnancy. Ginger should not be used where there is high blood pressure. Angelica and Benzoin increase photosensitivity.	**Vaporization, inhalations, aromatic baths.**
Colds	An infection of the upper respiratory system that causes nasal congestion and discharge, sneezing, headaches, watery eyes but *not* fever. It can be caused by a chill to the body. The illness is short-lived and dealt with easily by the immune system.	Expectorant, mucolytic, anti-inflammatory, balsamic.	Benzoin, **Cinnamon, Eucalyptus,** Juniper, Lavender, Lemon, **Peppermint,** Niaouli, **Pine, Rosemary.**	Cinnamon, Juniper, Peppermint, Pine and Rosemary should not be used during pregnancy. Pine and Rosemary should not be used by people with high blood pressure. Benzoin and Lemon increase photosensitivity.	**Vaporization, inhalation, aromatic baths.**

Condition	Description	Properties	Oils	Notes	Application
Coughs	A protective reflex by which a sudden blast of compressed air is released along the bronchial tubes and windpipe and through the voice box. Smoker's cough is a respiratory reaction to expel the accumulation of tar in the lungs. Coughing can also be a symptom of respiratory infection.	Anti-spasmodic, balsamic, expectorant, anti-inflammatory.	Benzoin, Cedarwood, Cypress, **Cinnamon**, **Fennel**, Lavender, **Pine**, Rose.	Cypress, Cinnamon, Fennel and Pine should not be used during pregnancy and Cypress and Pine should not be used where there is a high blood pressure condition.	**Inhalations**.
Hay Fever	A form of allergy affecting the lining of the nose, eyes and throat.	Anti-histamine, anti-inflammatory, calmative, anti-allergic.	Angelica, Benzoin, Camomile, Lavender, Lemon Verbena, **Marjoram**, Melissa, Neroli, Petitgrain, Niaouli.	Angelica should not be used during pregnancy. Angelica and Benzoin increase photosensitivity.	**Inhalation, vaporization**.
Influenza (Flu)	A respiratory infection caused by a virus. Its symptoms are chills, fever, cough, throat infection, headache, muscular aches and mucous discharge of the respiratory passages. It is a communicable disease which can be easily contracted and can be serious for the very young and the old.	Anti-viral, antiseptic, antibiotic, anti-pyretic, febrifuge, mucolytic, expectorant.	Angelica, **Cinnamon**, **Eucalyptus**, Ginger, Myrtle, Niaouli, Pine, **Thyme**.	Angelica, Cinnamon, Ginger, Pine, and Thyme should not be used during pregnancy. Thyme should not be used where there is a high blood pressure condition. Angelica increases photosensitivity.	**Inhalations** and **neat application** of essential oils applied to the lymph nodes of the neck during the early stages of infection.

Ailments of the Respiratory System *continued*

List of Ailments	Definition	Therapeutic Guide	Choice of Essential Oils	Contra-Indications and Cautions	Treatment
Laryngitis/ Pharyngitis	An infection or acute inflammation of the throat affecting the pharynx and the larynx, especially the vocal chords. It can cause the tonsils to swell, restricting swallowing, speaking and breathing.	Anti-viral, antiseptic, anti-bacterial, anti-inflammatory, soothing, analgesic.	Benzoin, **Fennel, Juniper,** Lavender, **Peppermint,** Pine, **Rosemary.**	Fennel, Juniper, Peppermint and Rosemary should not be used during pregnancy. Rosemary should not be used where there is a high blood pressure condition. Benzoin increases photosensitivity.	**Inhalations.**
Nasal Congestion/ Sinusitis/ Chronic Sinusitis	Characterized by mucous membrane inflammation of the sinuses caused by the common cold, constant and excessive mucus discharge from the sinus cavities, nasal polyps or an allergy such as hay fever.	Expectorant, mucolytic, anti-inflammatory, balsamic.	Benzoin, Cedarwood, Lavender, Myrtle, Niaouli, **Peppermint,** Pine, **Rosemary, Thyme.**	Peppermint, Rosemary and Thyme are not to be used during pregnancy. Rosemary and Thyme should be avoided by people with high blood pressure and Benzoin increases photosensitivity.	**Inhalations.**

Ailments of the Skeletal System

List of Ailments	Definition	Therapeutic Guide	Choice of Essential Oils	Contra-Indications and Cautions	Treatment
Arthritis	Inflammatory or degenerative changes causing pain and stiffness in joints. It may have	Anti-inflammatory, circulatory, analgesic,	Cypress, **Camomile, Fennel,** Geranium,	Cypress, Fennel, Juniper, Rosemary and Thyme should not	Localized aromatic massage on

186

	different causes as there are different types of arthritis.	vulnerary.	**Juniper,** Lavender, Pine, **Rosemary, Thyme.**	be used during pregnancy. Rosemary and Thyme should not be used where there is a high blood pressure condition.	the affected joints. Aromatic baths.
Backache	Occurs in different parts of the back and can be caused by wear and tear, occupational hazards, pregnancy or injuries. It can be due to problems affecting the inter-vertebral discs, ligament extensions and can cause muscle spasms. It can be very painful and cause severe restrictions in mobility.	Spasmolytics, anti-spasmodics, anti-inflammatories, nerve relaxants and analgesics.	**Aniseed, Black Pepper,** Camomile, **Cinnamon, Fennel,** Geranium, Ginger, Lavender, **Peppermint, Rosemary, Thyme.**	Aniseed, Black Pepper, Cinnamon, Fennel, Ginger, Peppermint, Rosemary and Thyme are not to be used during pregnancy. Ginger, Rosemary and Thyme should not be used when there is high blood pressure. Black Pepper can cause skin and mucous membrane irritation.	For the pain: **neat application of** Lavender to the affected area. Regular **aromatic back massage** and **aromatic baths.** If the problem does not improve, it means that an osteopath or physiotherapist may be needed.
Bursitis	Inflammation of the bursa, e.g. student's elbow and housemaid's knee.	Anti-inflammatories, analgesic.	Camomile, **Cypress, Fennel,** Lavender, **Marjoram, Rosemary.**	Cypress, Fennel and Rosemary should not be used during pregnancy. Cypress and Rosemary should not be used in cases of high blood pressure.	**Arnica ointment** with essential oils applied regularly, **aromatic cold compresses.**
Fractures	Aromatherapy can be an aid to recovery from fracture injuries and can be used alongside the conventional treatment.	Anti-inflammatory, circulatory, analgesic, lymphotonic, immunostimulant, vulnerary.	**Frankincense,** Geranium, Lavender, **Marjoram,** Myrtle, **Thyme.**	Thyme should not be used during pregnancy and is to be avoided with high blood pressure conditions.	**Apply blended essential oils** to the lymph nodes closest to the the fracture.

Useful Addresses

PROFESSIONAL AROMATHERAPY TRAINING COURSES

Nicole Perez
The School of Holistic Aromatherapy (SOHA)
108B Haverstock Hill
London NW3 2BD
UK
Fax: 020 7284 1315
e-mail address:
aromaschool@holisticaroma.fsnet.co.uk
Visitors by appointment only.

School of Holistic Aromatherapy (SOHA) and sale of essential oils in Japan
Hanae Kato MIFA
c/o Angelica
T & H Harmony IF
Kami-Osaki 2-9-26
Shinagawa-KU
Tokyo
Japan
Fax: 03 3449 5043

PROFESSIONAL MASSAGE COURSES

Linda Harness School of Holistic Massage
Swanfleet Centre
93 Fortess Road
London NW5 1AG
Tel: 020 7419 1325

PROFESSIONAL ASSOCIATIONS

The International Federation of Aromatherapists (IFA)
182 Chiswick High Road
London W4 1PP
UK
Tel: 020 8742 2605
Fax: 020 8742 2606
website: www.int-fed-aromatherapy.co.uk
Quarterly publication: *Aromatherapy Times.*

The Aromatherapy Council Organisation
PO Box 19834
London SE25 6WF
UK

The Institute of Complementary Medicine
Unit 15
Tavern Quay
London SE16 1PX
Tel: 020 7237 5175

The National Association of Holistic Aromatherapists (NAHA)
PO Box 17622
Boulder
CO 803 087622
USA
Tel: 888-ASK-NAHA
e-mail: naha@www.naha.org
Quarterly publication: *Scensitivity.*

**The International Federation of
  Aromatherapists**
PO Box 2210
Central Park VIC 3143
Australia
Website: www.ifa.org.au/index.htm
Quarterly publication: *Simply Essential.*

AROMATHERAPY PRODUCTS

Essential Oils
8–10 Mount Farm
Junction Road
Churchill
Chipping Norton
Oxfordshire OX7 6NP
UK
Tel: 020 608 659 544
Fax: 020 608 659 566
e-mail: sales@essentiallyoils.com

Index